17/6

14,B

SOME UNUSUAL
HEALING METHODS

by

LESLIE O. KORTH,
D.O., M.R.O., F.Ac.A.(Hon).

Author of
The Healing Sleep
Tensions a Practical Method for their Release
The Pyonex Treatment
Curative Hypnosis, Suggestion and Relaxation

A book of 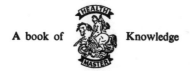 Knowledge

HEALTH SCIENCE PRESS
Rustington · Sussex · England

CONTENTS

	PAGE
INTRODUCTION	4
PREFACE	7
1. RESPIRATORY THERAPY (ON THE TREATMENT OF HIGH BLOOD PRESSURE AND HEART DISEASE)	9
2. THE CURATIVE POWER AND MAGNETIC QUALITY OF THE CULTIVATED HUMAN VOICE	16
3. SMOKING AND LUNG CANCER	22
4. CUPPING THERAPY	25
5. PSYCHROTHERAPY OR FREEZING TREATMENT	29
6. HOME OSTEOPATHY IN THE TREATMENT OF WHOOPING COUGH	32
7. HEALTH FROM YOUR FEET	35
8. FEET FIRST	39
9. BUNIONS AND HALLUX VALGUS AND THEIR TREATMENT	44
10. WHY EXERCISE!	48
11. REFLEX THERAPY	53
12. CHINESE ACUPUNCTURE	57
13. CHINESE PULSE AND MERIDIANS	62
14. HEALTH FROM SEA WATER	69
15. GARLIC, THE WONDER HERB	73
16. THE DISCOVERER OF IRIS DIAGNOSIS	76
17. UNEASY WAKEFULNESS	80
18. RHEUMATIC PAINS AND FEATHER BEDS AND PILLOWS	82
19. "EATING CAN BE A DANGEROUS HABIT!"	84
20. THE "WHY" AND "WHEREFORE" OF MASTICATION	88
21. THE PYONEX TREATMENT	91
22. STAMMERING AND ITS CURE	98
23. WHAT IT MEANS TO BE AN ADULT	104
24. THE RESISTING EGO	109
25. THE LADY WITH A GOITRE	113
26. THE MAN WITH AN OBSESSION FOR PLAYING WITH WATER	115
27. THE BOY WITH THE INTRACTIBLE COUGH	119
28. A COLD IS NOT AN ILLNESS	121
29. COLOUR THERAPY	125
30. HEALING MAGNETISM	129
31. THE PRACTICAL APPLICATION OF HEALING MAGNETISM	132
32. DISSEMINATED SCLEROSIS—SOME HELPFUL SUGGESTIONS	137
33. HEALING EARTH	143
34. EMETIC THERAPY	146

INTRODUCTION

By Denis Lawson-Wood, L.Th., Ph.D.

THERE are many ways of contemplating and assessing human beings and their activities. Individuals may be assessed in relation to their colour, creed or cultural environment; according to physique, athletic prowess, financial or social status, education, artistic gifts, and so on, more or less endlessly.

There is one way of contemplating not only mankind as a whole but also individuals; a way which seems peculiarly appropriate to modern times. One can focus one's attention on that aspect of man which we label the "scientific." It is a characteristic of man, distinguishing him from all other classes of life, that man has the ability to *know and to communicate*. This characteristic was called by Korzybski the "time-binding characteristic." It is in the light of this notion that I feel best able to build an adequate picture of the author of this present book and of his contribution to the cultural heritage of mankind.

It is in a special sense that I use the expression "scientist"; which special sense needs some elucidation.

In using the label "scientist" I do not refer merely to a technologist skilled in some special application, nor merely to one who is learned in one or more branches of "science," I refer to one who applies *scientific method*.

To a degree with which a person consistently applies scientific method in his thinking and overt activities he may be called "a scientist." This method is the one whereby a person seeks to know and understand natural phenomena and the operation of natural forces so that he may use and control these forces *with optimum predictability*.

The scientist, then, is one who observes facts, collects data, discriminates and evaluates the results of observations and experiences (his own and of others), and theories concerning them; and he arrives at some *tentative* conclusions himself. He then seeks validational evidence for his conclusions as soon as he can. He tests the soundness of his own conclusions, prepared to accept the outcome of his tests, whatever that outcome may be: in the light of these results he then rejects, modifies, retains, or forms new conclusions, which he again brings up for test as soon as he can. So the process goes on.

In my use of the label "scientists" I include the notion *"all of which is motivated by the highest ethic."* A scientist shares his

4

knowledge with others, thereby adding something to the totality of benefits available to mankind.

The author of this book, Leslie O. Korth, while still in his teens felt profoundly dissatisfied with medical treatment as he observed it being practised: for, he felt, it is not a sick individual that is being treated, but *the name of an illness*. Little or no attention being paid to the special way in which each person is ill; the whole focus seems to be on generalisations. If, for example, it was diagnosed "This person is suffering from influenza," symptoms a, b, c, d, e, f, g must be treated because those are the symptoms of influenza. If, by chance, he does not show symptom "e" then "because he ought (!) to have it but hasn't, the patient is wrong: and must be treated as if that symptom were present." Additional symptoms, simply because they do not come under the *general label* "influenza" tend to be ignored.

Mr. Korth, from earliest childhood years, had the desire to be a healer, a desire so strong that one can more fitly say "felt it as a Call." As soon as he began serious study of healing methods he realised that for him the direction would eventually have to be in conventionally "unorthodox" fields. He satisfactorily completed the requisite number of years study and training in well-established and generally accepted healing methods and disciplines. With this qualification alone he could have remained content to build up a prosperous practice. He was, however, not content to do so; and his whole professional life has been devoted to the search for ever better methods. He has come across and delved into a wide variety of healing systems, from all parts of the world, both ancient and modern and, whenever he has been able to form a *tentative* assessment that this or that method appears theoretically valid, he tested the validity of his conclusions by personal experiment, experience, and practical application.

The outcome of all this can be briefly summed up thus:— In Leslie Korth we have a versatile and experienced practitioner able to diagnose and assess the special needs of each patient, and then to select, from his extensive repertoire, the method to apply in this or that particular case likely to bring the maximum possible benefit to the patient. His aim has never been to prove the overriding superiority of one method over all others for all ills: his aim has always been that the patient shall be healed; and every effort made and method selected has been towards that goal alone.

In conformity with the scientific norms as indicated earlier, Mr. Korth has been ever ready to share his knowledge with others; and he has contributed much by way of lectures and papers to professional colleagues or contemporary practitioners.

I first met him when he attended a series of lecture-demonstrations which I gave on the Korzybskian non-aristotelian system,

General Semantics.   Since that first meeting he has, on more than one occasion, furnished me with information and material that has proved of inestimable assistance in my own research work and therapeutic practice.

In his "sharing with others" he has not confined himself within relatively narrow limits of professional circles: through articles in popular journals and magazines he has been able to extend his field of communication and influence to include a wide section of the general public.   This present work represents a selection of such articles, gathered together and published in book form.

Though, of course, this book can only represent a relatively minute fraction of his experiences and knowledge it, nevertheless, symbolises the man himself, considered as a scientist in the noblest sense of the word.

D.L-W.

Tunbridge Wells, 1959.

PREFACE

SEVERAL patients of mine, and others, who have read my articles, which have appeared from time to time in the various health journals, have been doing their best to induce me to have them incorporated in a book. I, however, shelved the idea, but it had evidently taken root in my mind, for I have now put it into effect, in that I have made a selection of those articles, which, so I believe, will be the most readable and, above all, the most practical in their therapeutic value. Some of them have been revised and amplified.

In spite of the varying intervals between the publication of each of the articles in the different magazines, and nothwithstanding that I did not entertain any thought of a possible relationship of one with the other, since they were written at different times, I have been able to group and correlate most of them so as to ensure some continuity, and yet each chapter is self-contained, which obviously has its advantages.

As "all roads lead to Rome," it is the earnest hope of the author that the reader will find in this book at least one "road" out of the many indicated that will eventually lead him to that beautiful State wherein health abounds; leastwise where some improvement can be attained.

Full acknowledgment is gladly given to:

Health and Life, Health for All, The Osteopathic Quarterly and Your Health (incorporated in The Osteopathic Quarterly), in which journals the articles were published, and which articles should now reach a far wider reading public in book form thanks to the Health Science Press in having embarked upon the publication and distribution of this work, to whom I am grateful for making this possible.

I am also greatly indebted to Drs. Ernst and Paul Busse, the joint authors of "Akupunktur-Fibel," published by Richard Pflaum Verlag, Munich, for granting their permission that their drawings of the "Chinese Clock" may be included in this book, see Chapter thirteen.

LESLIE O. KORTH.

SOME UNUSUAL HEALING METHODS

CHAPTER 1

RESPIRATORY THERAPY

(On the Treatment of High Blood Pressure and Heart Disease)

High Blood Pressure is one of the most prevalent complaints of the present day, and whilst not being a disease in itself it can be productive of many. Apart from somewhat alleviating the condition drug therapy is not the answer and it can make confusion worse confounded in the long run.

Both hypertension and hypotension are circulatory disorders, and as the breathing or respiratory centre in the brain is quite close to the circulatory centre it should now occasion no surprise for readers to learn that breathing has an enormous influence upon the circulation and hence upon the regulation of the blood pressure.

Now the vast majority of folk do not breathe fully. This vital function is reduced to something quite inadequate for the needs of their bodies and minds, through bad postural, dietetic and occupational habits. Added to these are the inevitable cigarettes. Most smokers inhale, so it stands to reason that the amount of smoke inhaled displaces that amount of life-giving air from the lungs, as well as poisoning the respiratory system. And adults are very shallow breathers as it is.

No food, no matter how dietetically sound it may be, can be properly digested without an adequate supply of oxygen. Is there any wonder then that there is so much digestive trouble and subsequent disease? The Torah (Gen. 2:7, 6:17, 7:15, 22, etc.) speaks of the Breath of Life; and quite apart from inhaling oxygen from the atmosphere the Yogi of India ages ago maintained that a cosmic Life-force is also taken into the organism at each breath, and this force is termed "Prana." It is a Sanskrit word meaning "absolute energy." Paracelsus had the same conception in his "vital fluid," and later Reichenbach called it "Odyle" or "Odic Force as a universal property of all matter in variable and unequal distribution." Still later there was Dr. Richardson, F.R.S., with his "Nervous Ether"; also Brunler with his "Biocosmic Energy," and there is to-day the X-Force of L. E. Eeman, further "discovered" and scientifically demonstrated by Dr. Wilhelm Reich under the name of "Orgone," which means "biological energy" surrounding and permeating everything. The Kahunas of Hawaii Islands gave the word "Mana" to this all pervading energy, which they used in the performing of miracles.

Since Yogi has been mentioned above it may well be stated here that the complicated exercises given in books on Yoga breathing are quite unnecessary for the purpose set out in this article on "Respiratory Therapy." In any case they should never be undertaken without a proper physical examination and instruction at the hands of a competent Practitioner.

Now to come back to our "muttons" as the French say: Of the ultimate cause of hypertension we know nothing definite. Various causes are mentioned. Of course, constitutional factors play an important role. Formerly one believed that the chief cause of hypertension lay in the capillaries being spasmodically contracted in an extensive area of the body, remaining in this state of contraction and thereby producing the increase in blood pressure in the whole circulation. Nowadays one believes that it is a matter of hypersensitivity of the constrictor centre in the brain, and this hypersensitivity is occasioned in the majority of cases by reduced breathing, a "chronic under-aerification." The normal stimuli of life, which are not registered by non-sensitive persons suffice with sensitive people to maintain the constrictor centre in abnormal sensitivity.

The diaphragm is the most important breathing muscle and separates the chest from the abdominal cavity. On inhalation the diaphragm descends, flattens itself out and thus increases the size of the chest cavity. The most powerful movement of the diaphragm takes place in the supine position, stronger than when standing or sitting. For all that, many persons are unable to breathe so well in the supine position and to satisfy their air hunger, because the pressure conditions in the thoracic and abdominal cavities are different on lying than on standing or sitting. Furthermore, on lying, the viscera press the diaphragm upwards more towards the head so that the lungs must contract more strongly. This is the real reason why with many heart sufferers the supine position is impossible. They suffer from orthopnea, i.e., they can breathe only in the erect position. Their air-need increases on lying, for only on sitting or standing can the diaphragm descend into the abdominal cavity, because the organs (viscera) no longer press against it.

The less flexible the thorax becomes with age due to shallow breathing over a lengthy period, the firmer it remains in the position of inhalation, and is no longer able to return to the position of rest; all the less also is the quantity of air that is exchanged on respiration. Therefore, people should be taught to prolong EXHALATION and to pay specific attention to this. To superimpose yet deeper inhalation movements upon the already fixed and firmly held inhalation position is incorrect, because such

10

efforts, which are in part erroneous and spasmodic, deepen the breathing only by a trifle on inhalation.

What is of importance is first to restore the flexibility of the thorax by prolonging the exhalation, and by the energetic movement of the diaphragm to relax the lungs better. The air exchange is thus promoted better than solely by the attempt to inhale forcibly. By such an attempt only the lung tissue which is permanently distended, becomes still more burdened, an excessive demand being put upon its elastic power. Hence it is quite wrong when some Physical Training Instructors cultivate only the inhalation, and decline to use the exercises by which the thorax is contracted and thus made smaller.

The activating cause of hypertension has been discovered in shallow, ineffective breathing. The outstanding symptom, viz., the considerable rise in the blood pressure, has been brought back to normal by correct systematic breathing exercises. And this is confirmed over and over again in one's practice. Also the subjective symptoms of this complaint are removed, such as the feeling of shortness of breath, sleeplessness, irritability, pressure in the head and on the chest, headache, palpitation giddiness, apathy to work, memory weakness. After three to six weeks of the breathing cure patients have become completely well without any other medicament, and have remained so as long as they continue to do the breathing exercises.

In order to remain healthy and capable everyone must eat and drink daily of sufficient quantity and quality. Hardly anybody will omit a meal, but there are always numerous individuals who just will not see that they must carry on with their breathing exercises day by day. Only those who indulge in sport regularly or sing daily need no extra breathing exercises. Among a hundred or so of professional singers examined in Munich not a single one of them suffered from high blood pressure. That speaks volumes in favour of correct, full breathing.

There is no doubt that the success of the cold water cure and of clay pack cures rests upon a strong stimulation, speeding up and deepening the breathing. But why not intelligently use the breathing apparatus that is part and parcel of the human organism and is thus constantly with us?

The first breath drawn in at birth fills the lungs with air—an amount of air which never disappears from the lungs. It is the so-called minimum air, that causes a lung, once it has breathed, to float upon water. To this air-quantity in the lung is joined another lot during growth and respiration that cannot be breathed away and disappears only then from the lung when the thoracic cavity is opened or the lung is removed from the thorax. It is the so-called "collapse air." Collapse air and the minimum air together form the residual air, which, as already stated, cannot be removed from the lung by breathing.

11

It has already been mentioned that the BREATHING centre influences the circulatory centre, both of which are close together in a part of the brain, and when the latter is not functioning as it should owing to the breathing centre not doing its job properly circulatory disturbances occur which later give rise to all kinds of disease processes. The condition can be corrected by properly regulated respiration, which must be carried out as follows:

Inhale slowly through the nose at the same time slightly protruding the lower abdomen which is then slowly retracted so that the ribs are lifted outwards and upwards towards the chest so as to fill the lungs *completely* with air, but without strain. At the completion of inhalation the breath is to be held for a second or two. Then—and this is another very important point to note, viz., the air is to be EXHALED through the mouth *on the sustained note of OO*. The lips must form the roundest possible O and the air must be exhaled slowly to the UTMOST limit, but again without STRAIN. This process is to be repeated for 10 minutes three times a day at first, working up to not more than 15 minutes at each practice a day, when the exercise may be done four times daily, the last one, it is suggested, being performed whilst lying in bed just before settling down for the night's rest; at other times in lying or sitting position; later in the standing position.

This respiratory exercise must be carried out every day with the greatest regularity, preferably immediately after a meal, as it will greatly aid digestion and bowel movements. The keynote to the success of this therapy, as it is indeed to anything else worth while, is PERSISTENCE, i.e., unflagging and regular application. To relieve the possible monotony of the sustained OO-ing sound, the OO-ing can take the form of a scale or tune.

If there be any blood pressure of a pathological nature present, then respiratory therapy will normalise it in a comparatively short time—and plenty of evidence can be adduced to support this claim —whilst a wonderful sense of well-being will be the lot of those who practice this respiratory technique: not only will the whole nervous system be revitalised, but the whole organism. Digestion will be improved as no food can be adequately digested without a full supply of oxygen, and this can be had only from the air we breathe. This fact warrants the repetition I have given it, and I also repeat here that one should be just as disinclined to miss one's daily practice of full breathing as one would miss a meal; but whilst feeding can well be dispensed with when ill to the patient's ultimate advantage, full breathing can but hasten the cure in those patients who are not too ill to practice it. In fevers Nature herself sees to it that the respiration is accelerated in order to supply the system with more oxygen to serve the increased needs of the organism as a whole.

So much has been written about diet that I am certainly not going to dwell on this subject here. I just wish to make a point

12

or two: Many thousands of people take much meat and animal protein with their meals and yet only a very small percentage get gout. But whoever has a disposition to gout can be saved from it if he carefully avoids all purines which bring about attacks of gout. Whoever feeds himself very modestly, taking no meat, and reducing the intake of protein and animal fat sufficiently, will not get gout in spite of the disposition to it. Similarly, with high blood pressure, whoever lives a corrective careful way of life will be protected from this complaint, even when he has the predisposition to it, for he will have excluded the various irritants and toxins without which, even when the predisposition is present, the complaint cannot develop—providing, of course, that the intake of oxygen is sufficient to deal with the food consumed, and this means habitual good, full, rhythmic breathing. Inheritance and the appearance of a disease on the one hand, cure and disappearance of it on the other, stand only apparently in contradiction, for a good Practitioner can, in spite of heredity, achieve success in the cure and maintenance of health of the one so threatened.

In order to explain the curative effect of deep breathing upon persons who are threatened with blood pressure, we must bear in mind that deep breathing on the whole can produce its effect in three different areas, viz., in the purely mechanical-physiological sphere by the change of the manifold conditions of pressure in the respiratory movement; in the chemical sphere that takes place in internal breathing, i.e., the giving up of the oxygen to the tissues and the taking in of carbonic acid gas—and finally in the purely nervous sphere.

A few words now on the efficacy of respiratory therapy in the cure of heart disease which was discovered by a Dr. Tirala of Vienna.

In recent years he has been most successful in opening up a new region of activity for respiratory therapy. It is not only with hypertensives that a large, flabby, dilated heart often occurs that causes the patient also a number of subjective complaints.

Palpitations, shortness of breath, a weak feeling, reduced efficiency, quick fatigue are symptoms that such a heart is considerably handicapped in its adaptability, as it is with changes in the heart musculature (myocardium) as with myocarditis and myodegeneration; further in all cases, which are due to so-called relative valvular faults; finally in all disorders which are due to poor, indifferent circulation of the heart muscle. All these hearts are treated with numerous medicaments, which, of course, are only so long "effective" as they are taken.

In the respiratory therapy as described herein not only have we a remedy in our hands to reduce these hearts, but to make them efficient once more. Whilst being misled by a mechanical conception, we have learnt that a really dilated heart can never again return to normal size. Dr. Tirala has been successful in a large number of cases, in proving, by careful X-Ray photographs, that the dilated heart could be made considerably smaller with the help of systematic breathing exercises. Naturally, the reduction depends on the reparative ability and regenerative power of the musculature. This one is unable to determine exactly in advance; only in the course of the cure will it become evident to what extent such a dilated heart can be made smaller. There have been reductions in the transverse diameter observed by Dr. Tirala of a few millimetres up to 4.5 cm.

The examination is conducted in the following manner: At the beginning of the cure an X-Ray photograph of the patient's heart is taken and the picture of the heart on the plate or film exactly measured. At the end of the cure, a second photograph is made, which is taken at the same hour of the day and precisely under the same conditions. The patient is directed with particular care to allow the exposure to be made in exactly the same position and with the same short depth of inhalation in front of the apparatus. One nearly always succeeds in attaining the same breathing position, which one can see from the position of the ribs and of the diaphragm very clearly in the pictures. Certainly, after treatment, the position of the heart on the diaphragm is mostly different; usually it does not lie flaccid any more; but the tone of the heart can be clearly seen from the outline. For enhancing the accuracy, cinematograph X-Ray pictures have been taken during the last 10 years, from which one can measure gross alterations of the heart with meticulous exactitude.

In none of the modern books on heart-therapy has Dr. Tirala been able to find even a hint about the therapeutic effect of breathing upon the heart. This latter is an important advance in the domain of heart therapy; for it is not only a matter of the heart "becoming smaller" as evidenced by X-Ray pictures and by palpation, but also of an appreciable increase in efficiency due to a genuine increase in the tone of the heart muscle itself. The exhalation-time which, in part, is a function of heart power, becomes considerably prolonged in the course of a few weeks with all patients. Patients who come with an exhalation time of 5 to 10 seconds, at times even only 1 to 2 seconds, learn not only to exhale correctly, but they acquire also the ability to exhale much longer, up to 30 and 40 seconds. This increase in the expiratory time goes together with a genuine toning up of the heart muscle.

Patients who complained of head pressure and giddiness and who were unable to walk any longer without having to stand at every 10 steps in order to take in a breath, report, not influenced by any suggestive questions, that they can walk again, that they are more efficient, that they have pleasure in going for walks and to wander about; in a word, that they feel themselves in possession of their powers. The feeling of strength, however, really depends upon the health and efficiency of the heart. Simultaneously with

14

the reduction of the size of the heart and its increase in efficiency the subjective feeling of well-being is enhanced.

But a note of warning here. Heart sufferers must not undertake respiratory therapy without expert guidance and supervision to begin with. Some patients may need a course of treatment to make good their biochemical deficiencies before they commence this therapy.

Dr. Tirala has had some amazing results, too, with his respiratory therapy in the treatment of other ailments, including sugar diabetes, dispensing with insulin injections in some cases, but let no diabetic sufferer act foolishly in this respect otherwise he may find that he has thrown out his means of survival.

Enough has now been said, surely, to convince the reader of the tremendous value of full, rhythmical breathing and of its wide scope in the treatment and cure of many hitherto intractible diseases.

CHAPTER 2

THE CURATIVE POWER AND THE MAGNETIC
QUALITY OF THE CULTIVATED HUMAN VOICE

NO MAN made instrument can ever match the exquisite beauty of tone and cadence of the natural, unspoilt or cultured human voice.

Now many ailments can be cured, alleviated, and what is of greater moment, prevented by voice culture, which, of necessity, involves full, rhythmic breathing; the very basis of good sound production. The use we put that sound to depends again upon the training in the correct use of the tongue and lips, and English people generally are woefully lazy in this particular respect, speaking through their teeth and mumbling their words.

H. G. Wells once said that "words are powerful things"; but how very much more effective is the spoken word when uttered by a free use of tongue and lips by a voice that is vibrant in its quality, rich in expression, making one fully conscious of the presence of a strong, magnetic personality, however soft or gentle is the enunciation of the words. There is indeed great POWER in words, not only in the actual words themselves but in how they are expressed. They can also be "tyrannous" vide Stuart Chase's unique book, "THE TYRANNY OF WORDS."

However, the acquirement of a good, resonant voice is not an easy matter. There are many hindrances and difficulties to be overcome, the removal of which constitutes a considerable part of the whole educative process in voice production. These manifest themselves in enervation and contraction of the vocal apparatus, with obstructive phlegm as a result of a catarrhal condition of the vocal chords in the larynx. In perhaps most cases it is a hidden catarrh of which most people are unaware. The result of singing exercises must serve to cleanse the affected, irritated mucuous membranes, as well as to regenerate and strengthen them, so that they can be made immune to any infection.

There are so many people, who suffer from catarrh, varying from acute catarrh of the throat to very distressing chronic bronchial catarrh. Constant associated symptoms are colds and susceptibility to atmospheric conditions. Such catarrh does not remain localised. It extends to the throat and nose. Below the larynx, catarrh of the respiratory passages or bronchioles or lung apices prepares the way for worse complaints. Bear also in mind the harm done to the voice by smoker's catarrh.

This catarrh cannot be separated from the condition of the voice, i.e., voice culture must include its removal and cure, or

16

conversely the therapeutic treatment must include the culture of the voice.

Many sufferers from catarrh are most dissatisfied that the nature of their trouble is not recognised. For example, a patient was operated on for a polypus on the right vocal chord; the beneficial effect of the operation, however, was not lasting in that later another similar one was indicated. However, the patient refused this to be performed, and rightly so, for a chronic catarrh had brought about the trouble in the vocal chords (weakness, fatigue, cramp, severe hoarseness). Voice culture dealt with the root of the trouble, so that the second operation became superfluous, and the patient has remained free from throat and voice trouble for very many years, whilst formerly he used his voice only with great difficulty.

In point of fact treatment by voice culture was not dreamt of, but its training was undertaken because of its aesthetic value.

Whoever had been ordered to take care of the voice by RESTING it, scarcely had the courage to trust a school which insisted upon the cultivation of the voice. It must be pointed out, however, that a curative result can not be brought about merely by singing of folk and classical songs or by participating in singing in a choir in spite of the fact that the organs of voice will thuswise be used. But it must not be overlooked that the voice will be used with all the inherent, acquired mistakes and deficiencies. To overcome these is truly a matter of voice production under expert guidance.

Voice inefficiency evidences itself externally by a long narrow neck with FLABBY musculature and FLAT chest. Another sign of a wrongly produced voice is the mouth being awry when speaking or singing.

The conventional suppression of habitually "clearing the throat" can only further conditions for catarrh. It should be indulged in whenever possible without, of course, causing offence to anyone.

In catarrhal subjects the chest tone, i.e., of deep, manly pitch proves loosening and healing, whilst the falsetto voice furthers the elasticity of the vocal chords, because of its high vibratory character.

One might mention in passing that in the culture of the voice age does not count. With the development of the voice the morale of the individual is raised. The exercises result in enhancing courage and energy where these are found wanting. The pupil gains quite a new attitude towards life. He has it in his own hands to foster this new state of mind by home practice.

Conscientious practice improves one's ability in sports of all kinds. While gymnastics and physical exercises usually train principally the extremities without appreciably altering the wrong use of the self, bad posture or flat chest not being thereby corrected, voice culture excludes all unnecessary and upsetting movements, so that an optimal effortless posture results of itself, as it were, and an enlarged "sports heart" need not be feared.

In Nature Cure, voice culture supplements or amplifies the treatment by light, air, water, heat, massage, dietetics, etc.

For the treatment of bronchial asthma breathing exercises have been known long ago. The asthmatic suffers periodically from difficulty in breathing because of a bronchial cramp, which hinders the expiration so that on inspiration a lifting up of the chest and shoulders takes place with the result that, in time, the chest and shoulders become "fixed." Medical science has produced a whole host of "remedies" against attacks of asthma, not only in the form of medicaments but also in technical respect, e.g., pneumatic chambers with varying degrees of air pressures. What the artificial difference in pressure tries to attain can be more effectively, simply and naturally achieved by the sufferer himself by voice culture.

It would appear that the fact is overlooked that the voice and speech of the asthmatic are very weak, and that being so one is unable to hit upon what ought to be the obvious idea that a strengthening of the larynx by work upon the voice would bring with it an improvement in respiration. The sounds produced extend their vibrations into the bronchial tubes and help in freeing their contraction. An asthmatic after some weeks' practice in voice production can effortlessly fill a large hall with his newly developed voice.

On the way to achieving this something important has taken place, viz., the secretion that previously could not be dislodged, is now loose, resulting in a great relief of the patient's condition. The one-time disturbed mucous membrane can now recover its normal function. The asthmatic learns to meet an attack whenever such is threatened and to hinder its development by exercising his voice.

Those asthmatics who have undergone training in voice production have reported a feeling of freedom, easier breathing, devoid of a feeling of anxiety and that the voice culture treatment was better than any medicine, raising the spirits to a joyful degree for the work of improving the vocal capacity exercised a strong influence in the way of inner release, which plays a role that is not to be underestimated, especially when psychological or neurotic conditions are present. Naturally for the achievement of the desired result there must be a readiness to persevere over a period of time. In those cases where the will to become well is lacking, and this cannot help but apply more to persons who have suffered from asthma for a long time, the prognosis is not so hopeful; but even here they must be persuaded to take up the exercises.

18

Similar good results are achieved in the treatment of emphysema. This lung distension can occur as an occupational disease. especially in glass-blowers and in players of wind instruments. The elastic tissue of the lungs becomes overstretched. But if voice culture is undertaken early, and the earlier the better, then the conditions can either be avoided or improved.

In passing it might be mentioned that the slowest breathing animals live the longest and are the least subject to infection. Nowadays it is not the practice to rest the lungs in tuberculosis as formerly, since Dr. August Bier indicated that rest in TB is likely to do more harm than good; but great care must be exercised. Sufferers from lung TB should not do breathing exercises on their own. They must submit to careful instruction in voice production by a qualified teacher, who must be made aware of the pupil's complaint, so that he can proceed with due caution.

Dr. Siegfried and Dr. Wohlfarth, lung specialists, have blazed a new trail by employing exercises for the voice in TB cases and have reported results of their cases at the Convention in Bad Kissingen, 1931.

After 10 years experience in two Institutions with men and women, Dr. Wohlfarth reported very convincingly upon the favourable effect of voice exercises on the breathing and circulation. When one succeeds in improving the voice and breathing and lung activity in general, then one is on the way to effect a cure.

As stated in my article on Respiratory Therapy, the circulation is dependent upon the manner of breathing. Voice exercises aid the flow and the distribution of the blood in the body, as well as the speedy elimination of carbon dioxide. Respiratory movements work on the circulation as a subsidiary pump, and thus, to some extent, lighten the burden of the heart. For example it can be observed that after singing practice the pulse rate of 88 before is reduced to 72, or, in other words, an obvious arhythmical pulse before the exercise beats regularly after.

In singing practice a pressure is exerted on the blood vessels of the head, and the sinuses are subjected to an increased air pressure, so that there is, besides an influencing of catarrhal conditions in the nose, ear and sinuses, a possibility of an improvement in the vision in short-sighted persons suffering from arterio-sclerotic changes in the eyes. This may sound incredulous. but it is known that even breathing exercises alone, without singing, have effected considerable improvement in the acuity of vision, and singing lessons have had the same, if not better, results.

We further observe an effect on the glands. The sweat glands are stimulated and people who never sweated could be bathed in perspiration on exercising the voice. In goitre a reduction of the thyroid gland can take place due to the improved respiration affecting the gland mechanically and relieving mental disturbances

There is also the possibility, in certain cases of advanced age, to achieve a more youthful voice. There is also the beneficial effect constitutionally.

In conjunction with the improvement of the bodily posture, fatigue symptoms disappear in a striking fashion due to the invigorating and refreshing effect of singing.

Not less impressive is the general change for the better; patients become more active, more communicative in an interesting way and complaints about their sufferings get less and less.

The psychological effect of singing must not be lost sight of either, as our mood at any given time shows itself so clearly in our voice reaction.

One patient, who always spoke in a loud, agitated voice, found an inner peace and increased concentrative powers through voice training. He was warned by his doctor some years ago that unless he acquired the habit of slow, deliberate yet easy speech with clear enunciation of each word, paying especial attention to the pronunciation of the final consonants of each syllable and word he would never lose his extreme nervousness and recover his health, which was seriously impaired at the time. He carried out his doctor's instructions. He underwent training at the competent hands of a professor of elocution, with the result that all his unrest, anxieties and inferiority feeling, together with his nervy, inarticulate, quick speech disappeared. His health was fully regained and his intellectual capacities were vastly improved which were also evidenced in his clarity of thought and reasoning powers.

Now I shall end this article on a personal note.

I became especially interested in the speaking voice when I, as a young man, was in Germany to acquire a knowledge of the language of that country, a language that is so involved and yet so thought-provoking.

Now, instead of taking lessons from a teacher of languages, who would have spoken German in his ordinary every day manner, I sought the services of a professor of elocution, who trained Germans in voice production particularly for the legitimate stage, which instruction embraced high-German (Hochdeutsch), correct pronunciation, enunciation, articulation, modulation and delivery, as well as breath control, of course. Thus I was able to acquire almost a perfect accent (which was also helped by my Welsh origin), and also an excellent command of the spoken word.

On my return to England a few years later, I received tuition in elocution from a London specialist as I had, and still have, a great love of the "speech beautiful." This specialist in the art of elocution was a great Shakespearean. He was a dwarf of a man, stunted in growth with a terrible spinal deformity due to a severe accident in early childhood; he was ugly in appearance but WHEN THAT MAN SPOKE he appeared to be indeed transfigured. His voice was deep, clear as a bell and having a rich resonance, with perfect modulation and delivery consistent with the dignity of the subject he happened to be dealing with at the time. Here truly was a magnetic voice of the very first order. No wonder Martin Harvey, who was once his adjudicator at the Haymarket Theatre, and who had the most disconcerting habit of sitting with his back to the stage, so I was told, was compelled to turn around towards the stage and exclaim, "What a voice; what a performance!" It was Macbeth.

There are different ideas on the methods of voice production, but perhaps the most revolutionary is the one described in Ernest G. White's book "SINUS TONE PRODUCTION." The author, if I recollect aright, maintains that the vocal chords do not produce the sound as is universally accepted to be the case, but that the chords are there for the purpose of controlling the breath, whilst the actual tone is produced in the sinuses of the cranium. The author puts forward very convincing arguments for his contention, and his book is well worth reading, and so is his "SCIENCE AND SINGING."

It is a thousand pities that this grand, dignified English language of ours should be so maltreated in every-day speech not only grammatically but vocally. Just observe some of the interviews on TV and on the sound radio. How one can suffer from discordant voices, inarticulate speech and bad grammar! And then we get plays the actors and actresses of which have mastered the art of good articulation, and it does not matter whether it be in dialect or in standard or Queen's English. But why confine this to the stage? Let us cultivate the beauty of speech and use it in our daily lives, and not be scared of consulting a dictionary over and over again in order to gain a command of words, and above all their intrinsic meaning. We should all be the richer in every way from such a study, and LISTENING then would become a real pleasure.

CHAPTER 3

SMOKING AND LUNG CANCER

QUITE recently I read in a German Health journal what a German medical specialist had to say on the subject of smoking and cancer of the lungs, and as I consider it to be of vital importance also to our English readers I feel it incumbent upon me to pass on the information here.

Dr. F. Lickint working in the statistical department of the State Hospital of Dresden-Friedrichstandt found that the number of deaths from lung cancer in the male rose by fifteen times from 1900 to 1955, by more than thirty times in the whole of Switzerland from 1905 to 1949, and by even more than forty times in England and Wales from 1899 to 1947. A similar state of things is to be found in the Soviet Union, in the Orient, in America and in other countries.

This enormous increase has made one wise to the fact that in many countries of the globe more people now die from lung cancer than from the formerly greatly dreaded disease of tuberculosis. Indeed, in the United States of America the yearly figure of deaths from lung cancer even exceeded the total cases of deaths from inflammation of the lungs and influenza. Cancer of the lungs, has, therefore become the most frequent cause of death of all the lung diseases.

In the search for one or more of the causes working in conjunction with each other, Dr. Lickint postulated eight outstanding points which have to be taken into consideration, so as to leave no doubt as to the real cause of such a rapid increase in lung cancer since the turn of the century. What now are these points?

1. As the increase in lung cancer was not observed before the turn of the century the exciting cause must have become active among mankind at that time or just before to an appreciable degree.

2. The active principle that produced cancer affected only males at first, and females later, and world statistics on lung cancer confirm this.

3. The cancer producing cause must affect all kinds of occupations, as with its increase not only intellectuals are attacked but also craftsmen and labourers.

4. The evil must be just as prevalent in the country as in the town as country folk fall a prey to it just as townspeople do.

5. On the other hand the substance that is responsible for inducing cancer cannot logically be present in those countries and in their peoples in whom an increase in lung cancer has not yet been observed.

6. The activating factor does not have any effect upon the animal world, especially upon our domesticated animals: dogs, birds, horses, etc., as up to now all these animals have remained practically free from an increase in lung cancer.

7. The substance to be found as responsible must, on close analysis, contain chemicals which are known as cancer producing, of which we shall hear more later.

8. Finally the proof that this substance is the cause would be enhanced if one succeeded artifically to produce a cancer formation with it in tests on animals.

The specialist now comes to the core of the matter without further ado in that he states that there is practically only ONE substance which fulfils all the eight conditions given above, and that substance is *tobacco* smoke in so far as it is *inhaled*. This drawing into the lungs is usually indulged in in cigarette smoking, which alone gives off an inhaleable mild sour smoke, whilst the smoke of a cigar or pipe has an alkaline reaction.

Before the inhaled tobacco smoke can act upon the lungs so as to produce cancer some thirty or forty years must elapse. This fact has been established by statistical data.

It comes to this then: A boy or girl, who starts smoking at about seventeen years of age will be afflicted with lung cancer (with few exceptions) at about forty-seven or fifty-seven years of age or later. In the meantime he or she feels generally quite well, and, therefore, does not pay the slightest heed to any words or writings about the danger ahead. Only in a certain percentage of cases does the so-called "smoker's cough" develop a few years before lung cancer manifests itself.

In all too many patients lung cancer is only then discovered after it has become well established when secondaries may be found in other organs, especially in the liver, in the skeletal system or brain.

Over the last few years it has been incontestably proved, within the framework of intensive analyses, that appreciable quantities of cancer producing tar substances are found in the smoke of cigars and cigarettes. *This fact must be especially emphasised, as even to-day it is maintained, in ignorance of the results of these tests, that no cancer producing substances in tobacco smoke have been determined.*

The analyses just referred to have been undertaken by numerous researchers among whom are Prof. Lettré and his co-worker Dr. Hahn of Heidelberg, Prof. Druckrey, of Freiburg, Dr. Seelkopf of Würzberg, the Englishmen Cooper, Lindsay and Waller of London, and finally, Dr. Lickint in collaboration with Dr. Buchner, Apothecary Pietsch and Dr. Brehmer.

Tobacco smoking over the years then creates conditions conductive to lung cancer, one of the conditions, not so far mentioned, being oxygen starvation in that the inhaling of the smoke must displace that amount of air commensurate with the amount of smoke inhaled, for obviously, the lungs cannot contain both smoke and the full complement of air at the same time. The whole organism is therefore deprived of its full quota of oxygen.

The mention of oxygen-lack reminds me of a gem of a little book, which a patient of mine brought back with her from a visit to South Africa. Its title is *"Oxygen:* Master of Cancer" by Frank Totney. He says that smoking interferes with normal, regular breathing, in that most smokers alter their breathing in some way whilst indulging in this habit. Smoking reduces the *free* oxygen in the inhaled air due to the burning of the paper and tobacco. Smoking clogs up the lung surface and thereby reduces the area through which oxygen could pass to the blood. Smoke is a suspension of very, very tiny particles in the exhaled breath. These tiny solid and fluid (tarry) bodies unfortunately stick to the lung walls to some extent, hence smokers' cough which is an attempt to shake them off again, in order to increase the useful lung area.

Young people are certainly not devoid of common sense, I therefore earnestly hope that what is written here will not go unheeded.

CHAPTER 4

CUPPING THERAPY

CUPPING, as it is called in English, is one of the oldest forms of therapy, and is very effective in the treatment of a variety of complaints. It is known in France as *"ventouse,"* in Germany as *"Schroepfen,"* and in America as *"vacuum"* or *"pneumatic"* treatment, and in these countries it is far more widely used by the medical profession as well as by the laity, more especially by the peasants on the Continent. As a matter of fact, I have in my possession an almost up-to-the-minute German medical publication on the subject, which goes to indicate that because a therapeutic method is considered "old fashioned" it should not, on that account be illogically discarded.

The Egyptians in ancient times used dry cupping in the treatment of disease, i.e., about five thousand years ago. Even in unexplored regions of darkest Africa it was discovered that the natives there used coconut shells to serve as "cups," which they applied to various parts of the body for curative purposes, whilst the Arabs in far off days applied the hollow horns of animals to the affected areas, and other races were found to use a hollow bamboo rod one end of which was placed on the skin with firm pressure, and the other end in the mouth. The air was then sucked up and a vacuum produced. After all, the oldest form of "cupping" is to be found in the mouth in that the lips are pressed on to the infected part and the poison, e.g., snake poison, sucked out. It is also thought that the saliva has curative properties, hence, for example, the dog *licks* his wounds.

About four hundred years before Christ there lived that great, enlightened physician Hippocrates who was evidently not slow to recognise the therapeutic possibilities of cupping. There were many other doctors of note in far off days who used the method, but in more recent times there was a French doctor by the name of Victor J. Junod who discovered, quite independently, the curative principle of cupping by observing the effect of atmospheric pressure upon the human organism as he climbed a high mountain. This discovery he employed in his practice, and the results he obtained from the treatment were so outstanding that they brought him early recognition by the French Medical Societies, whilst the medical schools of Italy, Germany and Austria warmly received him. There was also an English doctor by the name of Hadfield, who years ago, recognised the potentialities of this treatment in circulatory disturbances and diseases resulting therefrom.

We surely all know that an unhampered flow of the blood, which is itself chemically balanced and not surcharged with toxic matter, is the restorer and maintainer of health. Osteopathic treatment is of immense value in removing obstructions to this vital circulation of the blood and lymph, but unfortunately, for various reasons, not everyone can avail himself of the services of a qualified osteopath—indeed there may not be one in the area in which potential patients reside.

It is for all these that this article is written, for cupping treatment can easily be carried out by any member of the family in the home and prove a great boon. It can also be used as a most valuable adjunct by those who are attending an osteopath. Among the numerous complaints and diseases that can benefit from cupping are any painful congested area, bronchitis, asthma, pneumonia, pleurisy, boils, swellings, rheumatism, arthritis, and lumbago.

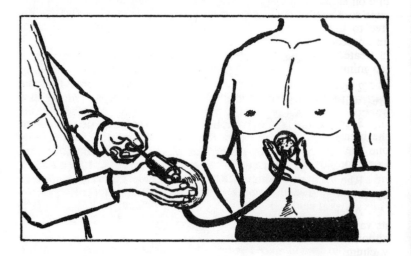

The *modus operandi* or technique is not difficult to follow. First of all obtain from any good chemist say a dozen of ordinary cupping glasses. They can be had in various sizes but a two inch size is recommended for the treatment of the back, chest and abdomen and smaller for the neck region. In order to create the necessary vacuum use a methylated spirit lamp. Hold the cupping glass with the opening downwards and place the lighted lamp slightly inside it for a few seconds, then very quickly apply the cup to the part to be treated. Cupping glasses can also be had with a rubber bulb on the top. This does away with the necessity of having the lamp, as the vacuum is made by first squeezing the bulb, then applying the cup to the skin surface with firmness and slowly letting go of the pressure on the bulb. The air in the cup will thus be sucked up into the bulb. To remove the cup just squeeze on the bulb again and lift. The best and most modern cupping glasses are now supplied with a suction apparatus in the form of a pump attached (see sketch). These have a great advantage over the other types in that the vacuum pull can be regulated, and they are made in all shapes and sizes so that they can be accommodated to the varying and unequal surfaces of the body.

For the general treatment of the spine, back, chest and abdomen or any soft structure proceed as follows:

1. *Spine and back.* The first cupping glass is to be placed over the spinous process as near to the neck as possible, the patient lying face downwards. The next is to be applied just below the first, and so on, right down the whole length of the spine. Then the cups are to be removed from above downwards and placed one on each *side* of the spine. This dual application will bring the cups to about halfway down the back. These must be left on for five to ten minutes, as indeed must the first lot. Remove them and proceed down in the same way until the lower half of the back is treated. They are to remain on this area for a further five to ten minutes.

2. *Chest.* Place as many cupping glasses on the chest as the area will hold. Let them remain there for five to ten minutes.

3. *Abdomen.* Place one cup on the solar plexus, just below the breast bone, then down on each side of the abdomen, placing one over the bladder region and one just above if there is room. Leave on for five to ten minutes.

Rheumatic pains in the arms or legs can very well be treated by cupping, and if regularly done results are most satisfactory.

After all the cups have been removed, take one and then in its vacuum state drag it firmly along the muscles of the back, chest, abdomen, etc., in all directions with sufficient pressure so that the vacuum will not be broken. This treatment gives the tissues a superb massage. It breaks down adhesions and thus removes hindrances to the circulation; witness the erythema or reddening of the skin, which the patient experiences as a most pleasant warm glow.

In order to ensure a good vacuum pull, care must be taken to see that the glass evenly contacts the tissue. This can best be done by applying, say olive oil to the skin. It also facilitates the "dragging" massage.

Slight bruising might take place in the treated areas, but this is of little consequence. Just suspend treatment for a day or so; otherwise treatment can be given every other day.

Finally, remember that as a prerequisite for sound, healthy functioning of body and mind, and for the restoration of health where this is lost, there must be a blood stream that is unhampered in its flow, and that the blood itself must be properly chemically constituted, but whilst the circulation can be improved by osteopathic and cupping treatment including cupping massage, etc., the right quality of the blood can be attained only by feeding upon whole, unprocessed foods, which have been grown upon soil that has been naturally manured, not an easy matter in these days of artificial fertilizers.

Other things being equal we are made or unmade at the table.

CHAPTER 5

PSYCHROTHERAPY OR FREEZING TREATMENT

THE WORD "psychro-therapy" sounds odd, does it not, at least the first half. It is derived from the Greek, and must not be confused with the word "psycho-therapy" as "psyche," also of Greek origin, means the soul, the mind whereas "psychros" means "cool." Psychrotherapy therefore signifies treatment by cooling, and the method used to achieve the necessary degree of cooling for therapeutic purposes, is freezing. This form of therapy can well come under the heading of hydropathy seeing that water in a solidified state may be used as an excellent freezing medium.

This freezing treatment appears to be little known and still less practised in this country outside surgery, but its efficacy is striking, not only in the relief of pain, but also in removing its cause viz: congestion, inflammation.

There is perhaps no better treatment than freezing in the manner to be prescribed presently for the alleviation of localised areas of pain such as lumbago, fibrositis, neuralgias, neuritis, migraine headaches, strains and sprains.

There are several freezing agents available, such as, to name only one, ethyl chloride, which is supplied in glass tubes each provided with a special spring nozzle, so that a jet of the solution can be directed on to the affected part until the skin whitens. But the safest and easiest for *home* use is ice in the form of ice blocks out of the domestic refrigerator.

LUMBAGO:

The method of application is simple. Let us suppose that father is suddenly striken down with an attack of lumbago, then mother or some other member of the family or friend has only to go to the refrigerator (comparatively few houses are without one these days!) and take out a few blocks of ice and put them into a basin.

Have the patient lie face downwards on the bed or sofa, then apply two or more ice blocks on the painful parts each side of the spine, but before doing so dip each block into a saucer containing ordinary common kitchen salt. Hold the salt covered surface of the ice block firmly on the affected areas with a towel in order to protect the fingers. See that a few cloths are placed under the patient so that they extend sideways over each side of the bed or sofa for the absorption of the drops of water as the ice melts when in contact with the warm body, thus preventing the wetting of the couch.

Very often only one such application suffices to effect the cure, but the skin over the region of tenderness must be distinctly frozen, so that the tissues under treatment present a whitened or parchment-like appearance, which can be ascertained by lifting a corner of the ice block and taking a peep. This frozen condition must be maintained for a minute or so, the time of application varying with the sensitivity of the skin, usually from a quarter to one minute.

Do you know that a burn can arise from ice remaining on the skin for too long a time? Care must therefore be taken that this does not take place. Should however, a burn occur then apply a lint dressing first smeared with either calendula or garlic ointment in preference to zinc ointment which I have seen advised. Fix the lint in place by adhesive plaster.

NEURALGIAS:

Freezing is a specific for all forms of uncomplicated neuralgia provided it can be done close to the site of the pain. If the neuralgia pain is situated at the lower part of the back of the head freezing along the painful path will relieve it.

Freezing is also effective in some cases of herpes zoster, i.e. shingles. Neuritis resulting from shingles is exceedingly painful and very difficult to eradicate by the usual medical measures and requires prolonged treatment, but it has been found that treating the condition by freezing brings about a speedy cure.

Neuritis in the arms or in the thighs and legs (sciatica) reacts most favourably to freezing, so does fibrositis or any other inflammatory condition.

COUGHS:

Freezing is not only very useful in allaying stubborn, persistent coughs, but is, happily also curative. Freeze each side of the upper spine including the neck region, where tender spots in these areas will be found on digital pressure. Migraine headaches respond well to this form of treatment, and certainly there can be found no better method for dealing with sprains and strains.

SPRAINS:

If an ankle or any other joint becomes sprained, spectacular results can be expected after freezing the painful parts. During and immediately after the freezing the joint must be kept moving. Little or no pain will be experienced and stiffness will be avoided.

Professionally the method can be used more extensively for example as reinforced freezing for deep seated pain due say to lesions at the exits of nerves and which are intractible to other forms of treatment. Reinforced freezing is effected by injecting sterilised water beneath the skin at the part to be frozen, or directly into the tissues until a marked bulging is produced, a freezing solution is then directed on to the protuberant part which causes a lump of ice to be formed under the skin or tissues.

It is said that "all roads lead to Rome, but I would add that some roads are much better than others, thus some therapies are better—more effective—than others, and freezing therapy ranks high among them for the complaints mentioned herein, freezing being of especial value for *home* use.

N.B. To prevent undue irritation of the skin after freezing all the salt must be carefully washed off the parts thus treated.

CHAPTER 6

HOME OSTEOPATHY IN THE TREATMENT OF WHOOPING COUGH

No PARENT or anyone else with feeling can possibly witness, unmoved, the fight for breath a child has to make when in the throes of a choking spasm occasioned by that intractible and most distressing complaint of whooping cough and the onlooker not being able to do anything to relieve the condition. All is well after the spasm is over, i.e., until another attack occurs, and another, and so on, for a long period of time. What a boon it would be for parents and others to know of a method whereby such spasms could be cut short or ameliorated!

Now, such a method I discovered in a German medical book I read some time ago, which was devised by a German doctor many years back, and which is very much akin to osteopathy as we know it to-day. This method comprises three alternative manipulations, either of which, so the doctor claims, can prove successful in cutting short the choking bout or at least lessening the severity of the attack and the total period that it usually takes for the whooping cough trouble to clear up—no mean achievement! The method can easily be learned by any member of the household, and even carried out by the victim himself, that is, of course, if he be not too young.

Of the three alternative methods now to be described, choose the one that you find most suited to your own particular aptitude, and to the child himself.

Method 1—Stand in front of the patient and firmly grasp the top of the ascending rami* of the lower jaw bone immediately below the cheek bone slightly in front of the ears with the forefinger and middle finger of each hand, placing the thumbs on the chin, and then pull the chin forwards and downwards strongly but with care.

Method 2—This manipulation is effected by hooking the thumb on to the lower incisor teeth, and with the rest of the fingers,

---

* *Each side of the lower jaw is roughly L shape, the upright branch each constitutes the ascending ramus (plural rami) at the top of which are two prominences, one of which articulates with the lower part of the temporal bone of the skull, slightly in front of the lower part of the ear, where movement can be felt in the joint by placing a finger there.*

grasping under the chin and then drawing the whole of the lower jaw forward and downward. The other hand is laid upon the forehead of the patient to effect a counter-pull. Naturally caution must be exercised not to exert too much pressure upon the teeth, but rather upon the lower jaw.

Method 3—In this method you stand behind the patient and position each thumb just above the angle of the jaw, then place the forefinger and middle finger of each hand on the chin and push the lower jaw downward and forward, or the fore-finger may press down on the lower back teeth to accomplish the same movement of the lower jaw.

As soon as any one of these manipulations is performed the child must take in a deep breath, and when this happens the spasm ceases at once.

The manipulation is so simple in itself that any reasonably intelligent mother, brother or sister, or anybody else who happens to be at hand at the time when an attack is on, can do it. It can be carried out without causing any further distress to the child, and once he has experienced the wonderful relief it is said to bring, he will lose no time in running to someone in the know as soon as he feels the cough coming on. It often is the case that even the youngest will try to carry out the manipulation on himself once he has experienced what it can do for him in the way of ridding himself of the spasm.

Whenever there appears to be much whooping cough about, parents and children should lose no time in practising these hand manipulations, for as it is claimed over and over again, the excellent results obtained by this simple method make the trouble in acquiring efficiency in it more than worth while, for after only a few seconds following upon effective manipulation the choking spasm is cut short, and the vomiting—a usual accompaniment of whooping cough—hæmorrhages and other complications which the increased blood pressure can produce do not occur. Even though the disease is not checked by the cutting short of the spasms, its duration will be considerably curtailed, and its character will be of a milder nature throughout its shortened course.

The doctor who devised the aforementioned manipulations explains their effect upon the choking attack as due, in the main, to relaxation of the neck musculature. The effectiveness of them has been confirmed in German medical journals, so I understand in which it has also been stated that sensible, older children, who have carried out the manipulations on themselves have invariably reacted well and at once, but of course they must be done by others for the very young ones.

The fundamental object of this manipulative procedure is to break the spasm while the child is compelled to take in a breath.

33

Another German doctor achieves this by this method. Have the child kneeling on the floor. Stand behind him with the right leg between the knees of the child; stretch both arms of the child upwards and grasp them with both hands, drawing the thorax upwards and over the slightly bent right knee, which is pressed against the child's back. Care must be exercised in carrying out this movement.

A small child may stand, say, on a stool. You are to stand behind him and place both hands, with the thumbs upwards, flat upon both sides of the child under his armpits; he is then to be lifted up and his shoulders drawn over your own chest backwards.

For those readers who might be uncertain about these manipulations it would, undoubtedly, be a good idea for them to ask their respective osteopath, should there be one in the district, to show them how the holds should be made and the movements done.

CHAPTER 7

HEALTH FROM YOUR FEET

IN MY London practice before and partly during the last war, I devoted the whole of my time to specialising in osteopathic treatment of the feet, the demand for which far exceeded the supply of hours available. This evidenced the dire need for such treatment and amply confirmed statistical data that three out of every five persons suffer some disability from their feet.

I was at that time, and have been since, much struck with the remarkable improvement that took place in the general health of patients which followed adjustments to the feet. They individually reported that headaches of uncertain origin had disappeared, digestive disturbances had cleared up accompanied by a feeling of the abdominal organs having been "lifted up."

All this was, in part, due to the altered posture that was brought about by the improved condition of the feet. Pelvic congestion was removed, and with the viscera better positioned, bowel action became regular and easy—with the result that long-standing constipation cleared up, and with this relief, haemorrhoids, too. Menstrual periods in certain cases were "automatically" regulated, and were no longer painful, whilst all kinds of incidental ailments disappeared.

So it was that I gathered from the conspicuous changes for the better in the general health of patients and from the improvement that took place in any affected organ or organs (as a result of skilled foot manipulations) that there must be some connection between the nerve endings in the feet and the proximal and distal parts and organs of the body. The study and application of Zone Therapy confirmed that the splendid results obtained were effected by what is known as "reflex action," occasioned by the treatment to the feet and by the subsequent change in the patient's posture, as already mentioned.

Zone therapy of the feet is a system of treatment that has been evolved by one Eunice D. Ingham, a member of the New York State Society of Medical Masseurs for influencing, through reflex action, the different organs and other parts of the body by very deep compression massage of painful areas found on the feet by digital pressure. This system is based upon the Zone Therapy of a Dr. Fitzgerald, who was at one time, a member of the Central London Nose and Throat Hospital. He enjoyed an excellent

35

reputation, his medical acumen being fully recognised and acknowledged.

Many individuals, who have no reason at all to complain about their feet will be greatly surprised to find that applying firm pressure to various small areas of the sides of the legs just above the ankles, to the soles and upper parts of the feet will elicit tenderness amounting, in many cases, to an excruciating pain.

Now, according to Dr. Fitzgerald and confirmed (by experience) by Eunice Ingham over many years, and by others working in this field (including myself) there are areas on each foot and on the adjacent parts which correspond respectively to each of the endocrine or ductless glands and organs of the body, which can be beneficially influenced by deep, heavy compression massage. This massage is done by using the fingers or thumb and making heavy, circular movements on the sore spot, wherever found.

These movements must be varied by upward and downward and sideways pressures. And one should make a practice of using this compression massage every day for five to ten minutes on each of the painful spots discovered; but should not treat all the painful areas at one sitting if there are many. It is better to leave one lot over to be treated on the following day, and so on, alternatively. Gradually these tender areas will clear up and the resultant improvement, which can be most striking, will not only manifest itself in the feet themselves but also in the general well-being of the body-mind.

Each gland or other organ can be beneficently influenced by this reflex-therapy. But a proviso must be introduced here, viz., there must be no actual bone displacement present. Should the painful foot condition not yield to compression massage as described above, then the sufferer should consult a qualified osteopath, who by virtue of his knowledge and skill will make the necessary adjustments should he find that these are required.

The immediate relief, in most cases, after skilled manipulative foot treatment, has to be experienced to be believed; but self-administered deep compression massage should never be neglected, even if only for the exhilarating effects that it produces.

As already stated, improvement and cures in any organ, gland, muscle, etc., are achieved by what has been called "reflex-action," a phenomenon that tends to establish the harmony of the vital forces within the body.

Here is an excellent example of reflex action which exercises a curative effect upon the affected part, although it may be remotely situated from the area of the foot under treatment.

Only a short while ago a patient complained of an acute pain in and around the nail of the forefinger of the right hand. This

36

finger was somewhat swollen and inflamed, and I diagnosed the condition as one of onychia, from which the patient had suffered for years, treatment of any kind being of no use whatever. The finger, be it noted, was too painful to treat directly, so I went to the corresponding toe, the second in the right foot, and there in the same area as that of the finger, I found an exceedingly painful spot on even slight pressure. Into this spot I inserted an acupuncture needle of silver. This little "operation" was scarcely noticed by the patient, and this greatly surprised her. After two minutes the needle was removed, and now, on pressing hard on the toe AND on the previously acutely painful finger the patient did not feel the slightest tenderness. There has been no recurrence of the pain, the thickening has disappeared, and with it the inflammation.*

This case alone will more than suffice to convince any person, not hard-bitten by scepticism, of the soundness of Zone Therapy by Dr. Fitzgerald, and of the efficacy of acupuncture discovered by the Chinese over five thousand years ago with the meridians along which the life energy flows, known as the Yinn and the Yang forces.

It would seem that the establishment of the balance of these forces can be helped by applying firm compression massage to those areas of the soles of the feet, and also on top of them, as well as up both sides of the legs just above the ankles and on their sides that are found to be tender or painful on digital pressure. But compression massage need not be restricted to the feet. It can be applied to other tender areas on any part of the body especially along both sides of the spine.

The healing effects which are so puzzling even to serious investigators of to-day, and which are so frequently brought about by the acupuncture treatment and nerve-point compression massage, such as that of Dr. Cornelius, sometimes instantaneously, find a possible explanation in the Chinese view, viz., that the skin can be looked upon as an extended "carpet" of the brain. This is a most intelligent observation on the part of the very ancient Chinese physicians.

Apart from the curative influence upon the organs and other parts, and of the body as a whole, which can be brought about by compression massage, the effect of this massage upon the feet themselves is excellent—removing crystaline deposits, adhesions and muscle tensions; and by restoring mobility of the joints of the feet by suitable manipulations of the bones, the circulation is greatly

---

* Please observe that NO substance of any nature is ever injected with the Chinese acupuncture; just a solid silver, gold or steel needle, especially made for the purpose, is inserted subcutaneously.

improved together with the nerve supply* so that the feet feel really alive with a delightful vital glow. One experiences an uplift both in body and in mind.

If this home treatment of the feet is conscientiously undertaken before winter sets in by those who have suffered from chilblains in the past, they can be assured with almost a certainty that there will be no recurrence of that trouble; and many other complaints can be ameliorated or averted by this practice.

---

* *Circulation and nerve supply always go together.*

CHAPTER 8

FEET FIRST

THAT this is an age of foot-consciousness is emphasised by the number of shoe shops which specialise in "correct" footwear. People generally seem to be waking up to the fact that foot troubles can produce many ailments in other parts of the body even far removed from the cause and which were formerly not suspected of having their origin in the feet.

Perhaps in no other region of the body can such accentuated pressure be found as in the feet, encased as they are in "coffins" during practically the whole of the waking life. The word "coffin" at once conjures up the idea of death, and most human feet are but half alive so far as their full function is concerned, as two out of every three people suffer from some form of foot defect with consequences so far-reaching that sufferers would indeed take more heed did they but know. They would surely see to it that their precious feet were put right, not merely by having the symptoms treated by the removal of corns and callouses, not by the wearing of arch supports, but by having subluxated bones adjusted and the feet rebuilt as a whole and then adopting proper shoewear and avoiding excessive standing and other strains on the feet.

To arrive at an understanding of osteopathic methods of foot correction let us first take a superficial glance at that marvellous structure, the human foot.

It is made up of twenty-six little bones, each most ingeniously shaped and articulated to serve the purpose of the whole. They are held firmly together by bands called ligaments, whilst the muscles and tendons, which give movements to the foot, add to its support and afford elasticity to the arches, so as to mitigate against the jarring of the spinal column. There are twenty-eight articulations or joints, and the foot has the ability to perform no less than one hundred and twenty-six movements. It has been stated that, according to engineering standards of measurement, the feet have to bear a stress of two hundred and fifty tons to every walking mile.

Some misunderstanding about the arches must now be cleared up. The foot has three arches: the inner longitudinal or spring arch, the outer longitudinal or weight-bearing arch and the transverse tarsal or instep arch. But what about that so-called arch that comes in for more attention than the other three put together, namely the much talked of "metatarsal" arch! Is it not true that a goodly number of assistants in the modern shoe shop will assure their customers that they have "dropped" metatarsal arches and will promptly advise the purchase of supports? (The question of arch supports will come up later). Here let us deal with that erroneous but prevalent idea of the existence of the metatarsal arch. One surely has no need to be thoroughly acquainted with the complicated anatomy of the human foot in order to recognise with very little observation that with all the heads of the five metatarsal or long bones of the foot in direct contact with the ground when the weight of the body is upon them, there can be found *no* arch, and to quote Dr. Hiss the well-known American Osteopathic Foot Specialist and Orthopaedic Surgeon, to ascribe an arch to the metatarsals is a misnomer.

Whilst granting that a support beneath and just behind the heads of the metatarsals certainly affords relief from pain and discomfort in certain cases of metatarsalgia, it cannot be corrective, as previously stated. The hollow or groove observed on the front of the upper part of the foot—especially in high-arched feet—certainly gives the appearance of the bones having "dropped," but that groove is really caused by the extensor tendons of the toes having become contracted, thus pulling them upwards in a hyper-extended position, with the end of the toes flexed so that they look like hammer toes without, however their fixity.

We now come to what constitutes the main cause of the majority of foot troubles, namely, shoes that do not conform to the natural shape or stress of the human foot. The whole economy of the foot is thus destroyed, and with complete lack of normal function or of very limited function malformation takes place in the course of time. True, there are shoes now on the market which conform to the natural shape of the foot, more or less, but what consideration has been given to the *stress* that each foot is subjected to?

Now a timely word about the wearing of arch supports, whether they be built in or inserted into the shoes.

Let us revert to the natural arches of the actual foot. We have already mentioned that the inner longitudinal arch is the *"spring"* arch, but if it be "dropped" it obviously has lost its spring, hence it follows that by placing a firm arch support—especially of the steel variety—beneath the arch, it certainly has the mechanical effect of forcing the arch upwards through the resistance caused by the weight of the whole body upon the foot. But, and this is the important point to note, the actual *cause* of the "fallen" arch has thereby not been touched. The spring or recoil of the foot is still absent and whatever slight recoil there may have been before, that "little" has now been taken completely away by the steel contrivance. The foot is now held in a far more rigid state creating further tension not only in the foot but all over the body as the sufferer goes stumping along, jarring the nerves of the whole of his spine at each step right up to his head, quite irrespective of whether the wearer experiences relief from the support or not. Hence, you see these "crutches" maintain and tend to worsen the very condition they set out to relieve, and this in spite of the fact that some foot sufferers are obviously relieved at first, whilst others suffer more acutely and discard them. Here is another point, the continuous wearing of arch supports must eventually weaken the muscles of the foot since the action of the muscles is restricted, and natural law has it that "what you do not use you lose." Further, the spring arch is so designed by Nature that it does not come closely into contact with the ground at each step and still less so when standing, depending upon the height of the arch natural to the individual. Thus, when pain is felt in the sole of the foot, it is due to the delicate nerves and blood-vessels being impinged upon; hence it can now be easily recognised how hard supports increase the pressure upon them and how "fallen" and particularly artificially supported arches enhance the disability, and interfere with circulation.

It is of interest to note that the osteopath finds the source of most foot troubles in the posterior transverse or instep arch, and this quite irrespective of whether the arch comes under the category of "high," "medium" or "low." The actual *height* of the arch has little to do with the pain experienced, except that, ironical as it may seem, the very high arch can cause the greatest discomfort if the alignment of the bones constituting the instep arch is affected by even the slightest displacement of the bones, although to all appearances the foot presents a perfectly normal shape. What can rigid arch supports do here where there is no prolapsed arch to lift!

If there be no pain or tenderness felt in ordinary daily life, *and none elicited when the foot is under examination by palpation,* then be the height of the arch what it may the foot of that particular individual is normal to him, so far as its function is concerned. "Comfort varies with function," says Dr. Hiss. It must be stated, however, that whilst a patient can be quite unconscious of any pain or discomfort in his ordinary daily activities, yet it *can* be elicited on palpation of the bones.

The instep arch is composed of four small bones named from within outwards, the three cuneiform (wedge-shaped) and the cuboid (cube-shaped). In a case of so-called "fallen" arch it is one or more of these little bones that have become displaced. Very frequently the scaphoid or navicular (boat-shaped) bone is involved too. The scaphoid is situated behind and is articulated to the three cuneiform bones in front, and if the normal alignment of these bones is disturbed, the arch is really more "broken" than "dropped," such "dropping" not being so much in evidence in high-arched feet. Thus the correction lies not in the wearing of arch

41

supports, but in the adjustment of displacements by manipulative technique.

It is indeed very remarkable how quickly most foot ailments will yield to skilled manipulative treatment; and not only do successful adjustments cause the pain to vanish but afterwards the whole body feels a wonderful sense of well-being.

While bad shoes are undoubtedly the major cause of many foot disorders, which must be corrected locally by manipulation of the feet, the osteopath finds that bad feet are also caused in many instances by structual faults elsewhere in the body. Such defects are largely traced to a lack of symmetry and balance in the bones comprising the pelvis and lumbar area of the spine.

The distortions found here are numerous and complicated and would require much space to describe. Briefly, the effect of these is to disturb the normal line of gravity falling through the body and to place an unequal weight-bearing stress through parts not intended to take such a stress. This weight stress can be deflected so that it falls too far forward, backward or to one side, thus straining the feet with every movement, and no matter how perfect the shoes are in time the normal relationships of the foot bones are disturbed. It is futile in these cases to attempt foot relief without prior spinal correction, because the foot distortion here is a compensatory effect. As in all other disorders, the osteopath primarily considers the body from the standpoint of the "whole," and while relieving distress locally he invariably seeks its cause throughout the entire structural mechanism.

A certain type of headache has often disappeared through foot adjustment. That awful dull and irritating ache in the upper back between the shoulder-blades as well as pain and tightness in the neck and the small of the back have likewise vanished. Patients report that organs that were prolapsed seem to have regained their normal position. This happy condition would automatically be brought about by the altered and improved posture causing the spinal column to straighten, and with this, lengthening of the spine and the uplifting of the abdominal viscera would take place.

This article would not be complete without a word of solace to the ladies lest they may think that by wearing "sensible" shoes they are doomed to deny themselves the adornment of what is styled a fashionable shoe with its smart high heel, which gives them not only physical but also mental uplift. Provided that your feet spend the major part of the day in low-heeled shoes, the wearing of high heels in the evening will do but little harm. After all you are then sitting down most of the time and, if you are at a dance, you dance on your toes anyway, though admittedly the high-heeled shoes do affect the normal alignment of the whole spine, so that to maintain a good posture an abnormal and great strain is thrown upon the respective muscles responsible for the erect state.

A good plan for you ladies to adopt is this, wear shoes in the mornings with little or no heels, a sensible walking shoe in the afternoons, and then indulge if you like in your high-heeled shoes in the evenings.

CHAPTER 9

BUNIONS AND HALLUX VALGUS AND THEIR
TREATMENT

WHAT parent who loves babies has not gazed with rapt admiration and with the tenderest feelings at the lovely little feet of his infant! Babies, with the fewest exceptions, are born with normal feet, feet that are as perfect in their design and structure as any artist could wish, having in them all the potentialities for their future correct functioning. What wonderful and beautiful little structures they are ! Soon—all too soon—they have to submit to the requirements of the modern age by becoming encased in shoes that neither conform to the natural shape of the feet, nor to the stress they have to bear, which, according to calculations made is no less than 250 tons, in the adult, to the walking mile.

The word "Bunion" is derived from the Greek and means "turnip." It is an inflammation and swelling of a small membranous sac which secretes lubricating fluid at the metatarsophalangeal articulation of the great toe. A distortion of this joint is usually associated with a bunion, which is accompanied by various degrees of pain, ranging from an acute type to a dull ache, depending upon the stage of the inflammation. It is really a form of bursitis and when it becomes infected it is then called purulent bursitis. There is thickening of the overlying skin covering this prominent joint.

The abuse meted out to the feet paves the way to these unsightly distortions, which are eventually brought about by the wearing of short shoes, narrow, pointed shoes, high heels and socks or stockings that are too short.

How many adults to-day can abduct, i.e. separate voluntarily the big toe from the second toe? Baby can, so can primitive people. How can one possibly feel happy with unhappy feet? Feet that should carry one through life without themselves suffering?

Although much has been said in the past about the evils that can arise from the wearing of high-heeled shoes, it must certainly be mentioned here in some detail that together with shoes with pointed toes—that other "civilised" abomination—they are the greatest cause of that ugly and often exceedingly painful distortion of the great toe commonly called a bunion. This distortion is, in point of fact, nothing more or less than a *Dislocation* of the great toe joint and is technically known as *Hallux Valgus*.

Let us now see what happens to the bodily posture of the wearer of high heels and pointed toes and the great strain that the organism has to contend with quite unnecessarily.

Were it not for the pull of the powerful back muscles the balance of the body could not possibly be preserved; but this 'pull' must make the wearer of high heels bend somewhat at the knees, cause the small of the back to take on an undue forward curve, and this exaggerated curve in turn causes the unsightly protrusion of the abdomen followed, in the course of time, by prolapse of the abdominal organs with its unpleasant sequelae. To compensate for this excessive lumbar curve the upper back takes on a rounded curve over and above the normal in this region, which results in drooping shoulders. To compensate for this again, the neck is thrust forward giving one the impression that the neck is trying to run away from the body. How these bodily changes can upset the economy of the organism can be left to the imagination.

At each step in walking the foot of the high heeled individual is jerked forward in the shoe with some force—especially in the court variety—is squeezed into the narrow part of the shoe, and, meeting with resistance, the repeated blows upon the end of the big toe cause the great toe-joint to buckle between the head of the great or first metatarsal bone and the base of the big toe. This is complicated by the malalignment and functional disorder of the *whole* foot.

A bunion can develop on the little toe. It is then known as a "bunionette" or "Tailor's Bunion," as it was at one time very prevalent in tailors due to their squatting upon their work-table with crossed legs, thus putting excessive weight or pressure upon the outer border or the little toes, which were constantly being rubbed on the table.

Usually a bunion is associated with Hallux Valgus, which is an outward bending of the great toe. What can osteopathy do here? Well, nothing so far as affecting a permanent reduction of the dislocation of the great toe joint is concerned. Nothing short of surgical interference can alter this condition. This is successful in some cases; but only in very severe cases where great pain and crippling are present do I advise patients to chance the operation. Some are gratified at the result, whilst others are not quite so.

In sufferers from bunions with hallux valgus it is found that other bones of the foot are also involved and these CAN be osteopathically dealt with and with success, so that as a result of the required adjustments the great toe joint itself is relieved of its former strain, always providing that suitable foot wear has been adopted by the sufferer.

With the greatly improved circulation of the blood, with the rehabilitation of the foot as a whole brought about by osteopathic

45

treatment, with the release of muscle tension and joint strain, the inflammation of the bunion soon subsides, and with the mobility that is restored to the joint the patient is freed from the discomfort, which can, indeed, be most acute. But although there may be greater mobility in the joint and the inflammation gone together with the reduction in the swelling, please note that the *deformity* as such still remains, and remain it will until surgically treated.

A helpful tip for home treatment of inflammation of a bunion is to soak a wad of cotton wool or a handkerchief folded into a pad in cold water in which three tablespoonfuls of Epsom Salts have been dissolved: i.e. to the pint of water. Squeeze or wring out and apply to the affected part. Cover with a thick piece of woollen material and keep this compress on all night. In the morning throw away the wad of cotton wool or wash the handkerchief-pad and apply the compress in the same way on the following and subsequent nights for a while.

The following, specially designed exercises for the feet may prove helpful.

1. Walk up and down a room on the outer edges of the feet, the soles and heels not touching the floor. To do this at the commencement it will perhaps be necessary to walk with bowed legs. This exercise should be done several times a day, without shoes or stockings, of course.

2. Raise the heels, the feet tiptoeing straight ahead: repeat this up-and-down movement for a few minutes several times a day. Endeavour when performing this exercise to rise on to the toes and lower to the *outer* edge of the feet, not allowing the inner side to touch the floor.

3. Sit on a chair with the feet raised from the floor. Bring feet upwards towards the knees and at the same time curl the toes towards the soles of the feet. Repeat this until tired: rest, then repeat as many times as possible during the day.

4. Same position as for number 3, but stretch the foot downwards, at the same time curling the toes upwards. Repeat as for number 3.

5. Feet raised from the floor, rotate the whole foot from the ankle inwards and alternately outwards until fatigue warns you to stop. Repeat as opportunity occurs.

6. Slow walking in a room, carefully observing that the feet are placed straight in front, Toe and Heel movement as in ballet walking i.e. the *Toe* is placed down first with the heel raised. Do not allow the inner side of the feet to touch the floor. If each foot can be placed directly in line with the other, as in the walk of the North American Indian, so much the better.

7. Stand with the feet parallel, i.e. close together, raise the toes from the ground keeping on the outer edge of the heel and part of the foot: repeat until tired.

N.B. After performing the above exercises bathe the feet in hot water with a handful of Epsom Salts added: then bathe in cold water for a minute. Dry thoroughly.

8. If the toes be flexed and extended to their fullest extent under water when lying in a full bath, this exercise of "wriggling" the toes will not only be more easily performed, but will also be more effective. Extension and flexion of the whole foot in order to mobilise and strengthen the ankle joint will be facilitated under water, and so will the exercise of the fingers and wrists.

CHAPTER 10

WHY EXERCISE!

THE title of this article is an exclamation and not a question, but if it had been put in the form of a question, "Why perform exercises?" it might well have been countered by another question, viz., "Why *not* exercise?" Is it not essential to discipline ourselves to the daily performance of physical exercises not only in order to become fit but to keep in good health? It is the purpose of this article to answer the question.

First, however, we must ask the further question, "What earthly good is it to go through a series of boring exercises at night, or in the morning, or at both times, when we use ourselves in a wrong manner every moment of our waking life in the way we sit, stand, walk and breathe?" To superimpose exercises upon habitual wrong use of the self only serves to perpetuate the wrong use and, what is more, aggravate the conditions responsible for it. Hardly any one of us knows how to stand, sit, walk or breathe as we should to ensure the maximum physiological efficiency. It is useless to try to teach correct posture or a system of exercise, whether for the direct purpose of achieving a good stance or for attaining general fitness, merely by telling the pupil what to do, or even demonstrating to him how a certain exercise should be done. He must first experience the *feel* of what is required of him, and he cannot gain this by mere verbal instruction. When we try to carry out instructions, nervous energy is bound to travel along those paths that have been established over the years in the use of the self, and if this use is not correct then the last condition may well be worse than the first.

How, then, can the reader learn to the best advantage to initiate the *brain* impressions that will enable him to improve his way of using himself, bearing in mind that without a new "sensory appreciation" the attempt will be a hit or miss affair? In this respect, there is nothing to equal Matthias Alexander's technique, in the application of which the pupil is made to *feel* the correct positioning of the head, neck and body. This is done by the guiding hands of the teacher, which gives the brain the actual *experience* of correct position. At first, the head and neck come in for the greatest attention, for, according to Alexander, the primary control of the whole body lies in the neck region, and mere verbal instruction cannot make the pupil aware of this. Alexander discovered this "primary control" by dint of concentrated and infinitely patient observation of himself in a mirror. The student of correct posture would be well advised to study Louise Morgan's fascinating book, "Inside Yourself" (Hutchinson, Ltd., 12s. 6d. net).

Much can be accomplished without the aid of a teacher, and later in this article certain methods will be described which will enable readers to acquire a new use of the self, which will be to their ultimate advantage in restoring and maintaining mental and physical health. All that is required is the determination to utilise the means whereby wholeness can be attained; these means are certainly not restricted to just one particular method.

Some years ago the writer came across an excellent definition of the difference between a natural strong man and a self-made strong man.

It was maintained that a natural strong man is one whose spine is in perfect alignment, and whose head is beautifully poised on his neck. This definition has been confirmed over and over again in the writer's osteopathic practice, in treating patients who have suffered an injury. Almost invariably, when the spine approaches the "normal," it is found that the possessor has a basically sound constitution and has always enjoyed excellent health.

The natural strong man, then, is one who happens to be blessed with what is known as a "straight" spine, and who unconsciously uses himself rightly in the way he sits, stands, walks and breathes, thus keeping his spine in proper alignment and causing no interference with his primary control. The self-made strong man, on the other hand, is one who, through the practice of strenuous exercises, has developed bulging muscles which are unnecessary for the promotion of good health.

In order to prevent this state of affairs, we should learn to "sit tall," "stand tall" and "walk tall," but always avoiding strain, except momentarily when stretching. Ideally, the seats we use should have no backs for us to lean against, but that may be asking too much to begin with. Furthermore the back of a chair may serve a useful purpose in that it can give us the correct "feel" to which we referred earlier. This feeling is conveyed to the brain, giving it what has already been termed "a new sensory appreciation," provided the following instructions are heeded :

On being seated at a table or at a desk, the chair should be drawn up as close as possible, so that the small of the back is in contact with the back of the chair. In this position, stretch the body upwards from the hips, then relax, taking care not to alter your posture and to keep your spine in close contact with the back of the chair. This posture will give a delightful feeling of uplift and a sense of ease. Try it! Breathing will also be facilitated, and digestive processes will be freed from the interference which arises when downward pressure of the abdomen causes cramping of the internal organs. The latter is one of the evils of a bad sitting or standing posture.

Generally speaking, the chin should be held slightly down and in, thus ensuring that the head is placed in the correct position in relation to the neck and the rest of the body structure— i.e. forward and upward.

An illustration which I have found to be most useful, particularly with children, in showing how the spinal segments may be separated from each other by an upward stretch, is to place one fist upon the other, keeping the lower one still and lifting the upper one slowly. Subsequently, when the hands are used on the person receiving instruction, he is able to "feel" what correct use is. It is amazing how quickly children respond to this practical method, for it enables them first of all to visualise the spine lengthening and then to *feel* it as they practise. It is possible to feel the forward and upward movement of the head if the hands are placed at the back of it, or, better still, perhaps, if the hands are clasped behind the head, pressing it upwards and forwards.

Now, all this requires perseverance, which, in turn, means discipline. After a surprisingly short time, however, great rewards will be forthcoming as new and improved habits in the use of the self establish themselves.

The foregoing procedure is more of a re-education in the art of using oneself to the fullest advantage than an exercise as such, and it is certainly a means to a wider end than could possibly be achieved by mere conventional exercises, which may be extremely boring. If one goes through the movements of throwing a ball without actually having one to throw, the "game" becomes tiring in a few minutes, whereas a similar game played with the real ball may be indulged in for a very long time without undue fatigue. The same thing applies if one goes through the motions of digging without a spade; it is all so purposeless.

We may believe that physical *jerks* (what an expression!) are "good" for us, but if they are practised out of a sense of duty, they do not evoke the enthusiasm that one puts into real games. However wrongly we may use ourselves in playing the latter, at least they are not boring, and as they are usually played out of doors we do get the benefit of the fresh air. Stereotyped movements are usually dull.

This does not apply, of course, in the training of athletes, for they have a definite goal in view and they work for it accordingly with healthy zest. Nevertheless, the athlete who has mastered the technique of primary control, and whose head-neck relationship is therefore correct, is the one who will excel in competitive races and games. For the ordinary person, however, the carrying out of the "daily dozen" is as unnecessary as it is soul-destroying.

It cannot be repeated too often that the right use of the self will provide the body with all the exercise it needs for its wellbeing. It has been observed that even wild animals, like the lion

50

and tiger, do not lose their strength, even in captivity, for the simple reason that they do not lose the instinctive right use of their bodies.

The psychological effect of "drawing oneself up to one's full height" can be immense, and this psychological and physical uplift may be perpetuated if the head is kept correctly poised upon the atlas, which is the first vertebra of the spinal column, on which the head is supported.

This entails re-education of the muscles that control the head and neck in situ, as well as in movement, for it is the imbalance of these muscles that is responsible for many local and general physical troubles, with their corresponding mental repercussions.

In order to relax the neck, lengthen the spine and broaden the back, one must continually affirm, "Head upwards and forwards," until the new habit has ousted the old and has become firmly established. In order that this injunction may be carried out in a satisfactory manner, however, it is desirable that the correct brain impression should be given by a teacher. If a competent teacher is not available, then the following procedure may be substituted.

Stand close to a wall without a skirting board, keeping the heels together and in contact with the wall. The back of the head should also be in contact with the wall, but if this causes the head to be tipped up and back, the chin may be grasped in the hand and pulled gently downwards and slightly inwards, causing the head to go upwards and forwards. This will produce a gap between the head and the wall, but this is of little consequence, since the head is now in the correct position. Wherever possible, observe the results in a mirror. When the correct head-neck relationship has been secured, wriggle the head and spine upwards so that the latter becomes fully stretched. Try to "feel" the neck spine coming away from the shoulders in the upward stretch; at the same time reach downwards with the arms and hands as though to grasp a couple of bags which you imagine to be on the floor close to the ankles, taking care, of course, not to look downwards. Further, imagine your feet to be firmly anchored to the floor, and then try to feel the entire spinal column coming away from the hip bones in the upward stretch. Relax immediately after performing this stretching exercise, *but do not alter the posture.* Now, on walking away from the wall, you should feel like a policeman who has been promoted, but without any of his rigidity.

The sitting posture is among the commonest acts which we perform, and there is no doubt that the oriental way of sitting is superior to that of the occident. For one thing, it prevents one from indulging in the pernicious habit of lounging, so wrongly beloved by Western peoples. Even if we continue to use the popular kinds of chairs and sofas, our manner of sitting may be

51

greatly improved to the benefit of our general health as well as our comfort, for although lounging may be very pleasant to begin with, it does not rest the body, nor does it aid the important digestive functions of the body.

Let us try the sitting position adopted by the Chinese. It may cause some discomfort at first, but, then, so does any other unaccustomed activity, until the muscles and ligaments involved have adapted themselves to their new use.

Three cushions will be needed. Kneel down, with one cushion under the knees, one under the toes, and the third under the buttocks so that it also covers the heels. Now, sit well back on to the heels, *keeping the spine erect* with the head poised easily on the neck. After some practice one will be able to sit in this position for a very long time, and instead of feeling tired there will be a feeling of exhilaration on arising. Using a low table, it is possible to write or type with ease in this position, while those who suffer from digestive disturbances will find it helpful to take their meals in the Chinese fashion. The same posture is useful for avoiding strain while watching television, reading, etc.

As an alternative, those who do not like sitting on the floor Chinese fashion, may use an easy chair and adopt a partial yogi pose, i.e. with the legs crossed. (The chair-arms limit knee-separation and so prevent the adoption of the full yogi pose). After the respective muscles and ligaments have adjusted themselves to the Eastern way of sitting, there will be no inclination to indulge in the slovenly habit of lounging. Correct posture, both in standing and in sitting, furthers bodily and mental processes instead of hindering them.

As Disraeli said, "The secret of success is constancy of purpose."

CHAPTER 11

REFLEX THERAPY

AT THE commencement of the twentieth century an English physician by the name of Henry Head discovered and disclosed a new method of diagnosis, which, most unfortunately, has largely faded into oblivion from the minds of the elite in medical circles; but which is now being revived especially on the Continent, so that it is sure of receiving full recognition in the perhaps not too distant future.

In the year 1889, Dr. Head showed that an important connection or association existed between the internal organs and certain spots on the surface of the human body. He stated (I now translate from the German):

"The sensitivity is not deep or only situated in the skin or subcutaneously. These sensitive zones have a definite relationship with the different diseased organs; but in many cases they (the zones) are far removed from the organs. The pain occasioned by the irritation is not brought about by any action upon the organ itself, for this latter can be a considerable distance from the sensitive surface area. Moreover, the sensitivity can be on the right side of the body, although the organ affected is on the left."

These tender areas, mostly elicited on pressure by the palpating fingers of the practitioner, are termed the "Zones of Head," and they are to be found all over the body. But, Dr. Head was by no means the first to throw light upon the connection between the surface of the body and the carefully guarded secrets of the inner organs of the human organism, and thus to find out the state of these organs. Long ago the wisdom of the Far East had already discovered this connection. Dr. George Soulié de Morant, a brilliant connoisseur and promulgator of Chinese medical knowledge, stated that the ancient idea of the relationship between the surface of the body and diseases of the internal organs goes far back as the late neolithic age.

The Chinese had discovered that a whole lot of points on the body surface were painful when an internal organ was disordered and that pressure on these surface-points caused the patient to feel an acute pain.

Also the Japanese in past ages had profited from the Chinese knowledge and developed it further. In A.D. 443 the Emperor of Japan caused physicians to come from Korea so that they could bring with them the Chinese teachings, and at the beginning of the seventh century a delegation of Japanese doctors went to China in order to acquire knowledge of the Chinese method of healing the sick and to bring it back with them to Japan.

Traces of the Chinese teachings can be found among other cultured peoples, e.g., the Arabs, Tibetans; but in the West little was known of these experiences.

It was only in the middle of the last century that a number of western doctors busied themselves with the reflex problem. In 1834, the founder of the Swedish Gymnastics, Dr. Ling, established that there was a painful spot present in heart disease on rubbing over the fourth and sixth dorsal nerves; and his school also discovered that there were definite areas of spinal tenderness or sensitivity in, for example, gastric disorders, these tender points being in the region of the sixth and eighth dorsal nerves on the left half of the body. Likewise in 1834 the brothers William and Daniel Griffin of America found that a connection existed between certain disease symptoms and certain areas of the spinal cord. It has been stated elsewhere that the theories of the osteopaths and chiropractors have been built up on the work of the Griffin brothers and of Marshall Halls, the osteopaths and chiropractors associating diseases of the organs with displacements of bones of the spinal column and other joints.

Dr. Abrams too found various regions on the body surface, which as the result of diseased organs, were acutely painful. He appears to have been the first to style such painful areas as "transferred pain." He treated them by "Psychro-therapy" (not to be confused with psycho-therapy) which is a treatment by freezing, either by ethyl chloride or some other freezing mixture, or by plain, small ice blocks covered with common salt. Another method adopted by this doctor was "Spondylotherapy" to induce a reflex curative action in an organ. This was done by concussion directly over the spinal segment involved or by percussion along side of it, i.e. on the transverse processes of the vertebra or vertebrae. Thus percussion on the transverse processes of the seventh cervical vertebra can effect a temporary lowering of high blood pressure, and if persisted in over a period may bring about a permanent improvement. Percussion in this area is also most useful in relieving spasms of asthma and angina-pectoris.

Another doctor to recognise the painful spots on the body surface as being due to visceral reflex was a Dr. C. Lange of Denmark in 1875. The appreciation of this fact, then and since, in diagnosis led to actual appropriate therapeutic measures which are happily proving so successful in our day, especially on the Continent.

A couple of years ago I obtained from Germany a book by Dr. Cornelius on "Nerve Points" (Nervenpunkte) formerly known as "Pressure Points" (Druckpunkte). In this work Dr. Cornelius describes the origin of these nerve points, how they arise, their

54

significance and treatment by reflex therapy. These nerve points are tender spots, varying in acuteness, and they can be found not only along the spine and on the back, but anywhere else on the body surface. Anyone who has undergone an osteopathic examination and treatment, as well as those who have received massage can unhesitatingly testify to the exquisite sensitivity of these particular spots on pressure being applied to them; but they have not been given the attention and treatment they undoubtedly merit simply because their influence upon the body welfare has not been appreciated. Before full health can be restored and maintained, these painful points must be sought for, treated and eradicated, either by the most effective method devised by Dr. Cornelius himself or by any other special technique which accomplishes this and which removes causes of symptoms by reflex action.

Cornelius was asked to describe his technique in a book, which he was most reluctant to do as you will see from what he writes (I now translate):

"When I now carry out the wishes from many quarters that I describe my technique, I do so with not too easy a mind. I hold the view that this extremely delicate technique cannot be learnt from the written word; but only by treating patients in a practical manner under the constant supervision of an expert. Without question there are a few who are gifted with a special sensitive touch which enables them to acquire the technique and who can find their way alone ... "

The first essential then to the practice of Cornelius's method is that the operator must have a most delicate sense of touch—a discerning hypersensitivity in the balls of the fingers. In some individuals this sensitivity of touch is inborn, whilst in others not so endowed, it can be achieved by practice, patience and experience provided they possess a "bent" in that particular direction.

It should be obvious then that this method (or any other for that matter) must never be undertaken by a practitioner, who has not thoroughly studied every aspect of the subject and acquired the necessary delicacy and skill in putting it into practical effect, as there can be unpleasant reactions arising out of the treatment, which must be understood and knowledgably dealt with accordingly. The ultimate result, be it soon or late, of this particular form of therapy can, however, be most spectacular, improvements and actual cures being permanent. After the object of the treatment has been attained, patients are urged to come for a periodical check-up and for further treatment should this be so indicated. This check-up should take place at least twice in the year, because the painful surface areas can recur in the course of modern living.

There are adverse factors and those we manufacture ourselves over which one does not exercise sufficient *conscious* control in dealing with them or in avoiding their occurrence. Neglect of these painful nerve points can lead to more or less serious illnesses. In any case they can be and are responsible for a lot of nervous tension and irritability. Where there is mental tension there is also physical tension; where there is physical tension there is an interference with normal bodily processes. One accepts the idea that it is necessary, or at least expedient, to seek the attention of a hairdresser or one's dentist at more or less regular intervals. Why then should one be indifferent to the possible therapeutic needs of the body?

It appears that the treatment releases pent-up energy confined within each surface spot that is found to be painful, from which, I venture to say, not a single individual is entirely free. The reflex action from the periphery of the body explains the unqualified success of osteopathy, the therapeutic effect of which cannot be wholly attributed to the adjustment of a vertebra or bone *as such*, but rather to the *reflex* action that is induced by the particular manipulation in a specific manner, according to the nature of the case, and influencing the organ involved, *via* the spinal segment under treatment. And here is an appropriate place to attempt to dispel a very prevalent idea which still exists in the minds of numerous members of the general public, that actual disease conditions cannot be treated by osteopathy, which they regard as a treatment confined to "misplaced" bones, strains, sprains and lower back pain, usually styled lumbago. In view of the foregoing explanation of reflex-therapy it should now be easier for those who cannot conceive of diseases being successfully treated by outward body manipulations, to become convinced that they can. There are, of course, exceptions, but even in those diseases which cannot be directly affected by osteopathy, suitable adjustments to the bony structure and osteopathic soft tissue-work on the skin, muscles and ligaments will so improve the nerve and blood supply especially to the affected areas, that considerable improvement in the general condition of the patient will be achieved so that his ultimate cure or near-cure can not only be facilitated but also hastened; but it is, of course a "sine qua non" that he must carry out the osteopath's instructions to change those habits of living that may be inimical to his full recovery.

CHAPTER 12

CHINESE ACUPUNCTURE

ACUPUNCTURE is a method of treating disease, which was discovered and used by the Chinese, in their great oriental wisdom, over five thousand years ago, i.e. three thousand years before Christ. The Chinese postulated that there are two vital forces at work in the universe, named respectively Yinn and Yang. Yinn has the attributes of the moon, viz. "silver," softness, femininity, also coldness, whereas Yang has the quality of gold, copper, warmth, strength, masculinity. When these two forces in the human are balanced in their flow of energies, in their respective directions up and down the body, through what is called their different meridians, perfect health exists and is maintained.

Disease develops owing to there being either too much Yang (over stimulation) present or too much Yinn (sedation). There is an imbalance of these two forces. In modern language we have "positive" and "negative." In the terminology of physiology we have the "Sympathetic and the Para-sympathic Nervous System," behind the functions of which may be considered the Yang and Yinn forces respectively.

The meridians just mentioned, of which there are fourteen in number, can be looked upon as "paths" along which these forces travel at lightning speed. They must not be confused with the anatomical nerve paths. The Chinese had diagrams of the human body on which they traced these Yinn and Yang meridians; along them points for treatment were marked. To-day, there are splendid modern wall charts. The best are by Dr. Stiefvater, one of the authorities on acupuncture in Germany.

This healing method finds support in an extraordinarily rich and ancient experience. The first of the early books on the subject in Chinese were translated into French and were published in France so far back as the 17th century and continued over the 18th up to the present day.

Acupuncture is now widely used by medical doctors in France; and German physicians, with their characteristic thoroughness have followed the example of the French doctors so that this form of treatment is spreading all over Germany. Their literature on this therapy is rapidly growing. I myself possess no less than seven German works on the subject, and it is from a careful study of these that I am able to use this valuable and effective therapy in my own practice. Unfortunately, there are no books on acu-

puncture printed in English so far as I have been able to ascertain.*
But encyclopaedias mention it.

What is the modus operandi of this therapy? Well, let us
see what the word "acupuncture" means: "acu"—sharp, pointed,
needle-like. (We have the word "acute" in English); "puncture"
is self-explanatory. Hence, acupuncture is a prick made with a
needle. Very fine gold, silver or steel needles are used, first on
the spots that are painful either spontaneously or on digital pressure, then on the different points shown on the meridians to be
influenced. The effect of the insertion of the gold, silver, or steel
needle or needles into these releases locked up energy.

Dr. Hunneke states that a short circuit is thus created, and
that with this release of energy pain disappears and the balance
of forces is established and the tone of the whole organism improved. Whatever the theory or the method may be, it assuredly
works; and in confirmation of this I shall now cite a case of acute
appendicitis which was cured in a most remarkable way. But
first let me say this, that although the very thought of inserting
needles into the skin may cause you to shudder, in spite of the
thousands of injections that are given almost every hour of the
day, you may take it from me as an actual fact that the many
patients whom I have treated experienced either no pain whatso-
ever, or only such a very trifling sensation as to make no odds.
They have no hesitation at all in having the treatment repeated
as many times as may be necessary, even asking for it because of
the excellent results obtained. And be it noted, no substance is
injected.

Now to a case of appendicitis treated by Dr. Neils Krack.

One winter evening he was called out to a nine-year-old youngster. The roads were so iced over that it was impossible for him
to use his car, and although it was only a short journey to the
boy's home it was also extraordinarily difficult and time consum-
ing to make it on foot. The doctor found the lad suffering from
very severe pains in the right lower abdominal region, with nausea
and vomiting. The pulse rate was 118 a minute and the temperature was 103. A point on the lower abdomen named "Mac-
Burney" was acutely painful on palpation, and there was also a
localised pain in that area.

There existed a condition of very acute appendicitis, the appendix being on the point of perforation, which, in the ordinary
way of things, ought at once to be operated on. However, the
hospital was 12 kilometres away, the roads frozen over so that no
transport was possible, and even if attempted would only have

---

* Since the above was written there has now been published by Health
Science Press the first English book on the "Chinese System of Healing" by
Denis Lawson-Wood, at 12s. 6d., plus 9d. postage with a foreword by Leslie
O. Korth, M.R.O.

added further danger to the patient. So what was to be done in the circumstances? The doctor, who had only recently become versed in acupunture, and, fortunately, had his set of gold and silver needles with him, decided to resort to acupuncture. He knew that the "appendix point" for acupuncture is to be found on the outside of the lower right limb, somewhat to the front, and about 3 to 4 inches below the knee, and that this part is painful only in appendicitis cases on digital pressure. The doctor inserted a silver needle subcutaneously and left it there for about thirty minutes.

During this time of sedation the slight tingling upwards caused by the needle subsided, the pulse rate was now reduced to 90 from 118 a minute and the temperature 99.6F. Pain had diminished to such an extent that the lad became cheerful. Next morning before surgery hours, full of qualms and misgivings, the doctor called upon his patient, only to find, much to his amazement, that the boy's bed was empty. He was out playing with his companions quite all right. No complications set in and there was no recurrence of the trouble.

Since the "appendix point" on the lower part of the leg is found to be painful on pressure *only* in acute and chronic appendicitis it takes on an important differential diagnostic significance. If the spot is painful on digital pressure then it can be taken that there is definitely an inflammatory diseased appendix. Sometimes the patient states that on pressure being applied to this point, there is also a sensation of pain in the region of MacBurney's point on the right side of the lower abdomen.

As we have already seen, during the treatment of acute appendicitis by acupuncture there occurs a lessening of physical pain, a dropping of bodily temperature and a reduction of the pulse rate, all of which indicate a reduction of the inflammation. Dr. Krack finds that a complete cure takes place by the following day. No kind of medicament is required, but a twenty-four hour fast supports the healing process.

Allopathic medicines and previous over-indulgence in alcohol can make the acupuncture treatment ineffective.

In cases of chronic or sub-acute appendicitis just one treatment will not usually suffice. This must be repeated at intervals of eight days. The painfulness or otherwise of the "appendix-point" on the leg provides the best indication for leaving off the treatment.

Attendant on such treatment one can see, after the local restoration, a general recovery of the patient, in that his bodily condition enjoys an all round improvement; there is an increase in his strength and in his functional capacity.

Taking all necessary precautions and using the acupuncture treatment aright many appendectomies can be avoided.

Dr. Krack, in the course of the last few years, has successfully treated by acupuncture about thirty-five acute appendicitis cases together with numerous chronic ones. After a successful treatment of a few acute cases he had them operated on later because of previously formed adhesions, but on these occasions no inflammatory signs of the appendix could be seen. Only in one single case did the acupuncture fail. Fortunately the severely inflamed appendix could be removed surgically in time before perforation took place. The cause of this failure was due to a great and long abuse of alcohol by the patient, and "fast" living.

Fantastic as the above citation may appear to be, I myself have proved the efficacy of this acupuncture therapy in appendicitis as well as in many other complaints.

A patient of mine for many years was a victim of chronic appendicitis, but he refused to submit himself to operative measures, notwithstanding the fact that no treatment brought with it any good results. Recollecting the acupuncture technique employed by Dr. Krack, I palpated for and quickly found the "appendix-spot" on the right lower limb. This point was acutely painful on digital pressure. I inserted a steel needle, which, believe it or not, the patient did not feel, and I left it there for thirty minutes. Shortly after the needle was in, the patient spontaneously stated that all nausea had gone and so had the great tension in the appendicular region on the right side of the lower abdomen; and with this release all discomfort disappeared too —there and then.

Another patient, this time a young lady, was in continual pain in the mid-dorsal region of the spine, which medical doctors, physiotherapists and osteopaths had failed to cure over the years. All my osteopathic efforts, too, were without any result, so I resorted to acupuncture. The result of the first treatment was spectacular, but it could not be and it was not expected that just this one treatment would suffice, having in mind the chronicity of the trouble. The pain returned, but it was now considerably less and the patient, of her own accord, asked for the needle treatment, as she had found it so effective and curative.

It may be asked—and it is a fair question—why doctors here in our own country do not use acupuncture in view of the splendid results achieved by doctors in France, Germany and other countries?

Most British doctors seem to fight shy of anything that is ancient in medical practice, but stripped of its mumbo-jumbo (which, after all, may not be mumbo-jumbo at all to the initiated) these ancient healers seemed to have had an intuitive wisdom that far surpasses so-called medical science of to-day.

Then again there appears to be no literature in English on acupuncture, and even if there were, the subject requires long, patient and assiduous study and an acquisition of a deftness in applying the technique.

There are also translation difficulties, in that the French medical specialists in acupuncture have had to make up their own terminology from the Chinese equivalent terms, which we here would either have to learn and adopt, unless we could establish an English terminology.

However, with a knowledge of either French or German, or both, British practitioners are not prevented from studying the authentic works of Dr. Soullié du Morant, Dr. de la Fuye, Dr. Niboyet and Dr. Chamfrault, in French; and those of Dr. Erich Stiefvater, Dr. Ernst Busse, Dr. Heribert Schmidt, Dr. Walter Lang (who wrote a book on acupuncture and the nervous system) and Dr. Broddle, in German. They could also study something written by the Japanese physician Prof. Dr. Sorei Yanagiya on Ein-Stich-Akupunktur (One Prick Acupuncture) which was published in German.

In conclusion of this great and complicated subject, I wish to dispel any impression that may have been conveyed by this article that acupuncture is the one and only therapy that can restore the balance of the vital forces in the body. Of course not; there are other alternatives, and neither this nor any other therapy can have more or less permanent beneficial results unless the WAY OF LIVING is such as to establish harmony in mind, body and spirit.

CHAPTER 13

CHINESE PULSE AND MERIDIANS

THE CHINESE PULSE

THE taking of the pulse rate and noting the strength of the beats have been, and still are important procedures for a long time now in medical practice; but this act is restricted to just one radial pulse located on the thumb side of the hand near to the wrist joint. It is helpful, diagostically, only in a general way, and is not related to any specific organ of the body, except the heart. The Chinese acupunture doctor, on the other hand, using the discovery of his very ancient forefathers, makes use of no less than fourteen *Radial* pulses, six of which are on the left and eight on the right, and these, in turn, relate to fourteen different organs, viz.: —

Left radial pulse:

1. Light pressure with 1st finger left hand : small intestine
2. Firm pressure with 1st finger left hand : heart
3. Light pressure with 2nd finger left hand : gall bladder
4. Firm pressure with 2nd finger left hand : liver
5. Light pressure with 3rd finger left hand : bladder
6. Firm pressure with 3rd finger left hand : kidneys

Right radial pulse:

1. Light pressure with 1st finger right hand : large intestine
2. Firm pressure with 1st finger right hand : lung
3. Light pressure with 2nd finger right hand : stomach
4. Medium pressure with 2nd finger right hand : pancreas
5. Firm pressure with 2nd finger right hand : spleen
6. Light pressure with 3rd finger right hand : three heaters
7. Medium pressure with 3rd finger right hand : circulation
8. Firm pressure with 3rd finger right hand : sexual sphere

To be able to discern the fine differences in the quality of each of the pulse beats in the six radial positions stated above, requires great sensitivity in the finger tips and much skill born of concentrated and patient practice. Diagnosis is arrived at not from the frequency of the pulse beats, but from their relative strengths. Such differences that are felt enable those, well versed in the art of pulse palpation according to the Chinese method, to relate them to the organ or organs affected. Thus the acupuncture physician can be made aware of any disturbance in the distribution of the life forces Yinn and Yang in one or more of the organs mentioned above. The meridan involved is then known, and the appropriate points on that meridan can be treated accordingly either by the gold and/or silver needles.

The fingers are placed on the radial pulse in the following order:

> 1st finger close to the wrist on the thumb side
> 2nd finger close to and above the 1st finger
> 3rd finger close to and above the 2nd finger

but the pressure, light, medium, firm, as directed above, must be exercised by only one finger at a time, starting with the first.

Some Chinese doctors and others, in their selection of the points to be treated do not primarily choose those that are painful on digital pressure, but rather do they first ascertain the energy-rhythm of the organism by the special method of observing the pulse as described above. These doctors believe that diagnosis can be made from the different pulse strengths making it possible to recognise changes in the respective organ or organs. They are then placed in the position either to cure or prevent disease, or at least to effect an improvement by acupuncture, using either the stimulating gold needle or the sedative silver or steel needle.

According to Dr. Stiefvater, physicians in Europe started, in the eighteenth century, to reintroduce in no uncertain manner, the observation of the changes in the pulse beats, other than their frequencies, whilst Dr. Johannes Floyer drew the first comparison between the European and Chinese teaching of the pulse. His observations referred to the pulse rate and pulse differences according to age, sex, way of life and time of day.

The pulse doctrine took a new turn when the Spanish doctor Solano de Luque had made new observations in regard to certain modifications of the pulse. Solano noted the double beating (dicrotous) pulse several times before the onset of nose bleeding. These observations led him to investigate the prediction of other bodily discharges, by means of the pulse. If the pulse is soft it indicates the occurence of strong urination; if it be hard then vomiting is about to take place. The longer the intermission of the pulse beats, all the greater is the "emptying" or discharge that follows.

Again according to Dr. Bordeu each disease of an organ alters the pulse beat in a specific way. One can readily see from this how closely his idea is related to the Chinese teaching of the significance of the pulse, and however fantastic this Chinese teaching and practice may appear, they cannot be brushed aside.

THE CHINESE CLOCK

Now, we come to a very helpful device, namely the Chinese Clock, for according to the hour that symptoms of a disease manifest themselves in diverse ways, the organ affected can be ascertained and the appropriate homoepathic remedies prescribed.

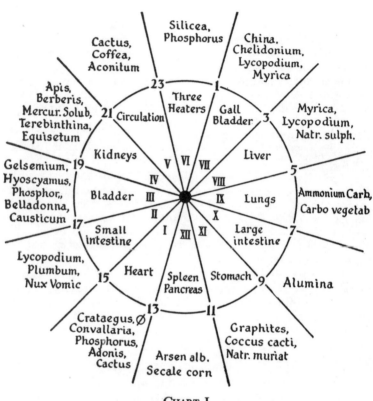

CHART I

CHINESE CLOCK

TIMES OF STIMULATION (TONIFICATION)

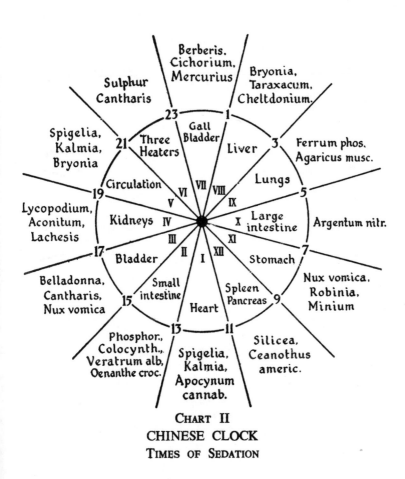

Berberis,
Cichorium,
Mercurius

Bryonia,
Taraxacum,
Cheltdonium.

Sulphur
Cantharis

Ferrum phos.
Agaricus musc.

Spigelia,
Kalmia,
Bryonia

Argentum nitr.

Lycopodium,
Aconitum,
Lachesis

Nux vomica,
Robinia,
Minium

Belladonna,
Cantharis,
Nux vomica

Silicea,
Ceanothus
americ.

Phosphor.,
Colocynth.,,
Veratrum alb,
Oenanthe croc.

Spigelia,
Kalmia,
Apocynum
cannab.

Gall
Bladder

Three
Heaters

Liver

Lungs

Circulation

Large
intestine

Kidneys

Bladder

Stomach

Small
intestine

Spleen
Pancreas

Heart

VII

VI · VIII

V · IX

IV · X

III · XI

II · I · XII

CHART II
CHINESE CLOCK
TIMES OF SEDATION

Let us go around this clock and pause every two hours to see what organ is involved:

Greenwich Time

From 1 to 3	...	...	...	... Gallbladder
From 3 to 5	...	...	...	... Liver
From 5 to 7	...	...	...	... Lungs
From 7 to 9	...	...	...	... Large Intestine
From 9 to 11	...	...	...	... Stomach
From 11 to 13	...	...	...	... Spleen-Pancreas
From 13 to 15	...	...	...	... Heart
From 15 to 17	...	...	...	... Small Intestine
From 17 to 19	...	...	...	... Bladder
From 19 to 21	...	...	...	... Kidneys
From 21 to 23	...	...	...	... Circulation
From 23 to 1	...	...	...	... Three Heaters

(Respiration, Digestion, Sexual sphere)

The above times are those of over-activity. Those below are times of under-activity.

From 1 to 3	...	...	...	... Liver
From 3 to 5	...	...	...	... Lungs
From 5 to 7	...	...	...	... Large intestine
From 7 to 9	...	...	...	... Stomach
From 9 to 11	...	...	...	... Spleen-Pancreas
From 11 to 13	...	...	...	... Heart
From 13 to 15	...	...	...	... Small Intestine
From 15 to 17	...	...	...	... Bladder
From 17 to 19	...	...	...	... Kidneys
From 19 to 21	...	...	...	... Circulation
From 21 to 23	...	...	...	... Three Heaters
From 23 to 1	...	...	...	... Gall Bladder

The attached diagrams show all the above at a glance, as well as the appropriate homoeopathic remedies, times of their administration and the organ for which they are indicated.

The organs of the human body are, according to the teachings of the Chinese, especially sensitive or receptive to various influences at certain hours of the day and night.

Should a disease condition evidence a worsening at any given hour, it can be concluded that that organ as shown on the clock diagram at that hour is affected even when no other diagnostic signs are present over and above those symptoms first complained of by the patient.

This hour of worsening is, at the same time, the hour in which the prescribed homoeopathic remedies will have the greatest effect, and these remedies need not be restricted to those stated on the clock diagram.

CHINESE MERIDIAN

There are twelve bilateral organ-meridians and two special ones, which traverse the surface of the body. In them flows the "stream of Life Force." By far the most of the Chinese treatment points lie on these meridians, and by treating these points the Chinese influence the flow of energy and thus centripetally influence the organs that are related to the meridians. These are:

1	Heart meridian	7	Gall bladder meridian
2	Small intestine meridian	8	Liver meridian
3	Bladder meridian	9	Lungs meridian
4	Kidney meridian	10	Large intestine meridian
5	Circulation and sexual sphere	11	Stomach meridian
6	Three Heaters meridian	12	Spleen-pancreas meridian

The two special meridians are:

(a) The back meridian, which extends up the spine from the coccyx over the centre of the scalp, down the centre of the forehead to the bottom of the upper lip.

(b) The front meridian, which extends downwards from the chin through the centre of the front part of the body to the centre of the pubic bone.

These latter two are not related to any organ. They represent a special closed circuit of the circulation of the Life Force, but are related to the other meridians.

It is interesting to note that Dr. William Fitzgerald at the time he founded ZONE THERAPY did not appear to have had any practical or even theoretical knowledge of the Chinese Acupuncture, yet there is a very vague similarity of his lines of force to the meridian paths discovered by the Chinese. Dr. Fitzgerald's Zone Therapy seems to embrace the same principles, so far as conduction of the Life Energy is concerned, as are embodied in the meridians of the Chinese. His pressure points, however, bear no relation to the painful spots on the body tissues or indeed to the meridians themselves.

Instead of gold and silver needles used to elicit reflexes the doctor employed digital pressure mostly on the toes or fingers. Small tightly fitting rubber rings are also used to exert the required pressure.

He divided the body into ten zones, each zone extending up the body, back and front, from each toe. Zone one extends up the front of the centre of the body through the right half of the nose and over the scalp. Zone two extends up from the second toe; zone three from the third toe and so on up to the fifth or little toe. The same applies to the five toes on the left half of the body, so that the ten zones' lines cover the whole of it both back and front. Similar lines are drawn from the fingers of each hand which join, at the shoulders and neck, those coming from the toes of each foot. The pressure is applied to the toe (or finger) of the zone to be treated, and this latter is determined by the nature of the complaint.

There are other points of pressure. For example to alleviate a stubborn cough the forefinger is to be pressed down quite hard in the hollow just below "Adam's apple." To relieve one from nervous strain the hands are to be folded as in prayer and the interlocking fingers squeezed as hard as possible for a few minutes at a time. This helps anyone in an awkward or unpleasant situation not requiring the use of the hand. I understand, as a matter of fact, that the Chinese were the first to use this method.

The attention of the medical world was drawn to Dr. Fitzgerald's discovery of Zone Therapy. It was pointed out that compression massage and pressures on certain zones did restore physiological functioning in those regions of the body that are affected, irrespective of their remoteness from the part being actually treated.

This zone therapy cannot be dismissed with a scornful shrug of the shoulders as humbug, much less so the acupunture of the Chinese, for Dr. Fitzgerald is a professional man of no mean repute. He was a member of the staff in the Central London Nose and Throat Hospital. He was, too, assistant to Professor Politzer and to Professor Otto Chiari, whose medical text books are so well known in the world's medical circles.

What this Life Force actually is we just do not know, but it has been very clearly demonstrated by the experiments of Baron von Reichenbach and by others active in this fascinating field of research. Reichenbach gave the name of "ODIC FORCE" to the LIFE ENERGY, but the name is of no consequence. What does matter though is to KNOW that such a power exists, and that it can be used for the great benefit of the health of mankind.

CHAPTER 14

HEALTH FROM SEA WATER

NOT so long ago a remarkable scientific treatise on the "Pharmacology of Sea Water" by Dr. Weiss was sent to me from Germany. It is a very comprehensive work, and is compiled with characteristic teutonic thoroughness. No pains seemed to have been spared in the extensive research that has been made by numerous German doctors as to the curative properties of sea water, with its all embracing chemical constituents, and also its richness in trace-elements such as gold, silver, copper, etc., so essential for the normal functioning of the body, and without which life could not be sustained. There is an imposing set of tables, and the literature that has been consulted on the subject extends to over three hundred medical authors.

It was about sixteen years ago that I first became acquainted with the therapeutic value of drinking sea water. It was then that I came into possession of a large tome on NATURHEILKUNDE (Nature Cure) by a Dr. Brauchle, and this is what this medical man had to say about the consumption of sea water.

Hippocrates and the ancient Egyptian physicians have all recommended the drinking of the water from the ocean for the purpose of cure, and in the history of medicine one will find physicians continuing to advocate this method, and who make mention of its therapeutic value. Here follows a summary of what is most important:

Nutriment is only wholesome when it contains all the essential materials conducive to maintaining health. If the composition of the soil is faulty, then the food cultivated upon it will also be lacking in mineral salts. Therefore, such deficiencies should be made good by the drinking of sea water.

The ocean is a collecting basin of all the important mineral salts. Life had its origin in the sea itself and right up to the present day the cells of the animal and human organisms are bathed in blood, whose serum in its composition, reveals a remarkable conformity with that of sea water.

So much, on the one hand, have diseases due to vitamin deficiency been investigated—so little, on the other hand, do we know what harm is caused by lack of mineral salts, or by wrong combination of these salts. Yet it is pretty certain that diseases due to faulty metabolism and glandular troubles, also many forms of tuberculosis, nerve condition, anaemia are all caused by deficiences in the mineral salts. Also cancer appears to be orginally related to this lack.

69

The drinking of sea water in correct dosage will provide essential material imperative for life, enhancing the power of resistance and immunity to infectious diseases, and it will increase the healing tendencies as well as the general capabilities of the individual.

Through the strong alkali reserve, which sea water has, it reacts upon over-acidity of the body, e.g., rheumatism and gout. Medical observations have proved that the whole organism can be toned up by the consumption of sea water. Catarrh of the alimentary tract, of the gall bladder and of the liver, intestinal stasis, chronic constipation, *hypochlorhydria and hyperacidity of the stomach juices are all favourably influenced by the internal use of sea water.

The drinking of this water is not only effective in the treatment of the diseases mentioned above, but is also appears to be strikingly effective in the treatment of all skin diseases. In support of this I cannot do better than translate the case history of a Dr. Ruzicka, Professor of Hygiene, which gives an account of this doctor's own astonishing cure of an intractible skin disease from which he suffered for over thirty years : —

"The critical condition of left leg, which four years ago led me seriously to consider having it amputated, was as follows:

The skin of the calf was surrounded by red eruptions, a condition known as lichen, which is a papular inflammation of the skin, of thirty years duration, that had defied all kinds of treatments. This presented a severe local appearance of an otherwise 'wandering' skin eruption over the whole of the body, which was very troublesome accompanied by itching, bleeding and festering skin patches.. An unexpected, sudden turn of events brought about a change in this tragic drama, which had such a poor outlook for me, in that, without any relation to the bad leg I underwent a regular, general cure by the daily drinking of sea water. And, wonders of wonders! After a week, I noticed a striking lessening of the itching and, partly, also of the hyperaemia, and then later the erruptive rash receded more and more in a most remarkable manner and to such a degree that I feel quite well again as if by a miracle after thirty years. The extraordinary effect of the sea water evidences with great certainty, that my trouble was a deficiency disease conditioned by the lack in my system of substances found in sea water."

Thus it would appear that sea water contains practically all the "Biochemic remedies" "rolled up" into one single medium.

However, care must be exercised in its administration in accordance with the nature of the case to be treated, and especially the particular patient who is undergoing the treatment must observe his reactions, as sometimes unexpected side-effects are experienced.

* *deficiency of gastric hydrochloric acid*

These, however, are rare and are generally looked upon as a "healing crisis" which eventually lead to a cure. But not everyone can tolerate sea water in the same way. Side effects may take the form of stomach cramps or diarrohea or some other constitutional disturbances. In these cases the dosage—more of which anon—is to be reduced until complete toleration is achieved. It is desirable not to exceed the toleration dose of sea water in these cases.

The sea-water-drinking-cure achieves its fullest effect only by keeping to a certain diet which should consist mainly of

1. raw vegetables in the form of salads and fruits
2. foods rich in vitamin, such as whole meal products, etc.
3. milk and milk products, yoghourt, little or no meat.
4. no ordinary table salt must be taken. Flavour with sea water.

The duration of a sea-water-drinking-cure is several months. The success of the cure will be hastened and enhanced when ordinary table salt is completely avoided.

It is inadvisable to exceed the prescribed quantities of sea water, as this is likely to slow down the curative process.

The cure is to be conducted in accordance with the following régime.

Sea water is to be taken on an empty stomach first thing in the morning, then at 4 p.m. and again last thing at night. It is desirable to dilute the sea water each time with eight teaspoonfuls of mineral or tap water.

DOSAGE. 1st and 2nd weeks; 2 tablespoonfuls diluted as above three times a day.

3rd to 7th week; 3 to 7 tablespoonsfuls thrice daily diluted.

From the 8th week onwards; 8 tablespoonfuls thrice daily diluted.

Should the increased quantity not be well tolerated then the patient is to revert to the next lower dose, but without interrupting the cure.

DOSAGE FOR CHILDREN. Up to 2 years of age; $\frac{1}{4}$ of the adult dose.

From 2 to 10 years $\frac{1}{2}$ of the adult dose.

From 11 years on; Adult dose.

Whoever, for some reason or another, is unable to continue with sea water drinking, he can then use sea water in the cooking instead of ordinary salt. Sea water can very well be added to soups and salads. Sea water, however, should never be BOILED.

In regard to diabetes Dr. Bensch reported in 1949 that patients had repeatedly stated that after drinking sea water they had no need to keep to the formerly prescribed diet for this disease, because the sugar content in the urine had diminished and eventually had cleared up completely, and they felt physically fresh and better than ever as the result of taking sea water.

To sum up then: Sea water should be taken in the doses mentioned, but before drinking it, it would be advisable to pass it through a Berkefeld filter, obtainable from any chemist.

It has proved effective in the following diseases: stomach and respiratory disorders, tuberculosis, circulatory and metabolic disturbances, such as diabetes, nervous conditions, disorders of the uro-genital system, kidney complaints, all skin diseases, rheumatism, gout, and it is helpful in cases of cancer. Salt water applied as compresses is a great cleanser and healer of sores, wounds internal and external ulcerations, and is very comforting and beneficial in cases of external cancers, e.g. of the breast.

It may be of interest for readers to learn that there is a firm in Bremen, Germany whose business it is to send ships well out into the Baltic sea for the purpose of collecting sea water from the depths of the ocean for bottling and distribution to hospitals and nursing homes for therapeutic use.

CHAPTER 15

GARLIC—THE WONDER HERB

(This article is based upon information derived from a German Source).

THESE days a great deal of publicity is given to the so-called "wonder drugs"; but as unforeseen detrimental side-effects become apparent and prove most disconcerting to those of the medical profession who use them, the qualifying word "wonder" loses its potency. Not so, however, with garlic.

The excellent effect of this wonder herb has been known by folk medicine for a very long time. Its splendid therapeutic reputation is extremely old. Garlic is mentioned no less than twenty-two times in the medical prescriptions of the Egyptian Ebers Papyrus 2000 B.C.

The workmen who built Cheops' pyramid over a period of many years received garlic regularly in their food on the advice of Egyptian physicians.

From the 12th to the 17th century it certainly could not have been omitted from any book on herbs.

Only in the 19th century did the doctors cease to consider it to be an essential remedy. As against this view, however, the French Academy of Science in Paris recommended the use of garlic in 1925 as a preventative against arterio-sclerosis. It is considered that the main sphere of use of garlic is in the calcification of the arteries and in high blood pressure.

As long ago as 2000 B.C. (Ebers Papyrus) it was employed in intestinal complaints, an indication which holds good right up to the present day, and this is confirmed by modern pharmacology.

Loeper, Marcorici and Leclerc recommend garlic in acute and chronic dysentery and intestinal catarrh. Roos recommends it for pin worms and Leclerc for maw worms, especially in children.

E. Meyer looks upon garlic as a specific where there were symptoms of nicotine poisoning. Smoker's catarrh and diarrhoea are due to nicotine indulgence. The beneficial effects of garlic in diseases of the respiratory tract have been written about by various authors.

In bronchial catarrh and emphysema garlic facilitates breathing, and in T.B. of the lungs it aids expectoration. Minchin is of the opinion that garlic has even a kind of specific effect upon

Koch's tubercle bacillus. Also its good effect upon gangrene of the lungs is reported by four French doctors.

Leclerc maintains that garlic is a prophylactic against influenza.

Such a variety of indications is really astonishing and it is worth while to summarise the beneficial results of garlic: it reduces blood pressure, it fosters digestion and elimination, it purifies the blood and controls diarrhoea.

One may well begin to ask what are the constituents of garlic that bring about such far-reaching beneficial effects!

Garlic certainly does not stick its "light"—or should I say "odour"—under a bushel! The odour is caused by the oil of garlic, which is volatile and a product of decomposition of the sulphur-containing glycoside alliin. Also worthy of note is the fact that the constituents of garlic are also bound with organic iodine, which hastens the metabolism of the body, speeding up the exchange of cells that have become inefficient in their function. It also lowers the viscosity of the blood.

Furthermore, garlic is rich in secretin, which stimulates the secretion and elimination of the glands. Thus are its disinfectant, bacteriological and antiparasitic properties explained. It rids the body of intestinal parasites (pin and maw worms) and of the minute germs of dysentery, typhoid and paratyphoid, and influenza; and it even enhances the defences of the body against cholera.

The action of garlic upon the digestive system is described by W. Kretschmar as follows:

"Garlic is passed to the bile from the stomach via the liver. It stimulates the secretion of bile, concentrating itself in the gall bladder. At the same time it stimulates also the other digestive ferments, thus intensifying the whole of the digestive process. Finally, garlic exercises a favourable influence upon the intestinal flora, which enhances the resistance of the body to disease bacteria such as typhoid, dysentery, etc."

The favourable action of garlic upon the circulation (it is a prophylactic against high blood pressure, calcification of the arteries of the kidneys) is due to various causes. For one thing garlic restricts disease putrefactive processes in the intestines and facilitates the movement of the blood in the body, which could otherwise be upset by such intestinal toxins. Furthermore, garlic distends the small arteries and capillaries, and it appears to enhance the energy of the heart. It is even included in the latest publications in the group of mild heart remedies.

The favourable action of garlic in diseases of the upper air passages is due to its loosening and liquefying properties, also its ability to improve the circulation of the blood as well as to its attested bactericidal power.

Wasiky showed experimentally that a very high dilution of garlic oil, viz., 1 : 50,000 acted restrictively on the development of proteus bacilli, whilst with the powerful disinfectant phenol a much stronger concentration, viz., 1 : 400 is necessary to achieve the same result.

These many-sided and changing effects of garlic seem to explain the fact that cancer diseases very seldom occur where a considerable amount of garlic is consumed, i.e., during the whole of a person's lifetime.

Possibly the various intestinal toxins, which are removable by garlic, possess cancer-inducing properties.

From what has been said it will be seen that to-day, and in the past, garlic can be considered to be a genuine remedy; but like every other remedy it must be prescribed individually, as it can act in an irritating and harmful way when taken in excess. In this respect Lohner, for example, warns against the use of garlic compresses and enemas containing strong garlic when treating infants and small children for worms, as very severe ulceration can be caused.

As a spice it suffices to use garlic sparingly. *Too much* of any *good* thing is bad.

CHAPTER 16

THE DISCOVERER OF IRIS-DIAGNOSIS

EIGHTY years have elapsed since the discovery of Iris-diagnosis by Dr. Peczely, and readers of this book—yes, even those who have gone into the subject of iris-diagnosis more thoroughly and enriched it with valuable observations and new discoveries, know very little about the discoverer himself and of his life and work. Therefore, it will certainly prove of interest to our readers to bring before them a faithful portrait of the discoverer, Dr. Ignaz von Peczely.

An eventful and fruitful life began in the year 1826 in Monyorokerek, when Ignaz von Peczely, son of an estate official to Count Johann von Szechenyi, first saw the light of the world. The young lad drew attention to himself even in the tender years of childhood through his intellectual capabilities. Then, while a scholar of the Premontreer Grammer School in Szombathely he carved such perfect figures out of wood, with the aid of a simple penknife, that the then Prince-Bishop von Gran Scitovsky wanted to send him to Rome for further instruction. When one takes into consideration that Dr. Ignaz von Peczely displayed those gifts at the early age of thirteen years (gifts which later led him to his discovery of iris-diagnosis) one can easily comprehend the manysidedness that Peczley manifested in his later years.

In the year 1838 he accidentally wounded an owl in the wing. He lifted up the wounded bird in order to take it home. However, the owl buried its claws in his right hand with such a rage that the boy, in trying to get free from it, fractured the owl's right leg with his left hand. Both glared into each other's eyes. In that instant, when the leg broke, a little mark of blood appeared in the right yellow eye of the owl which remained as a dark mark after the healing of the broken bone. After this observation the boy quite forgot the whole incident.

After finishing at the Grammar School he was trained to be an engineer. In 1848-49 he fought as first lieutenant in the Hungarian War of Liberty, was twice wounded and was decorated for his bravery by Ludwig Kossuth himself. After the suppression of the War of Liberty, Peczely was interned in Koposvar, where he, having lost his former situation with the Count Szechenyi, was compelled to earn his living as a dancing and fencing master. In 1851 he received an appointment as gymnastic and drawing instructor at the Koposvar Grammar School, and remained there until 1853; and at this time produced the very successful self-portrait which was cherished by his family.

Up to the year 1860 he followed his original occupation and worked as an engineer. In the years 1858-60 he made his first acquaintance with homoeopathic remedies at the home of a relative, Dr. Gulyas, who was a homoeopathic doctor in Kaposvar. A year later he returned to his parents in Egervar, Com. Vas., taking with him the most common homoeopathic medicines: aconite, arnica, belladonna, bryonia, phosphorus, pulsatilla, silica and sulphur.

When an employee of the Court Estate became seriously ill with fever, pain in the chest, cough and haemorrhage and no doctor at hand, Peczely's mother, whose most cherished wish it was that her son should choose a medical career, begged him to prescribe his remedies. Peczely gave aconite, bryonia and phosphorus every half-hour alternately. When the doctor did arrive in a few days, the sick employee was well. At this time a girl with cancer was also brought to Peczely, and he gave her sulphur and silica, and also in this case recovery followed the treatment. Thereafter the news quickly spread that Peczely was a "wonder-doctor" and soon there came a great pressure of patients from near and far who would not be held back until they were brought before him.

Then it was that Peczely made various observations and wondered why all these people had different coloured eyes and why there were different lines, dots and marks to be seen on the anterior surface of the iris. From then onward he paid great attention to the human eye.

One day there came a man who had a conspicuous mark on the right eye. As Peczely was looking at the mark, the line in the eye of the wounded owl suddenly occurred to him. He made a test and asked the patient whether he had not suffered an injury to the left shoulder. After receiving an affirmative answer he further examined the man's eyes and saw that on a point of the iris corresponding to the hour of six o'clock, there was also a mark which he had seen in his owl so many years ago. To the question whether he had not also fractured the right lower limb, the patient again replied in the affirmative. Thereupon the thought came to Peczely that injuries to the body left traces behind in the iris. From this day on, which may be looked upon as the day of discovery of eye-diagnosis, Peczely examined the eyes of every patient.

Soon he built up a system, in that he endeavoured to explain all marks in the iris through clinical findings. This is how he himself spoke of it:

"So I observed at first various kinds of light and dark spots and discolourations on the anterior surface of the iris. I then looked for the similar illness having corresponding marks, and conversely again to discover the same mark relating to the same sickness. After a short time I began to relate to each patient the past history of his surmounted illnesses."

Naturally, after such a "wonderful" discovery the number of patients grew to such an extent from all parts until at last the authorities stepped in and prohibited Peczely from treating the sick any longer. However, at this time he recognised that he was born to be a doctor and wished to become one officially, and in the Spring of 1862, in his 36th year, he matriculated at the University of Budapest as a medical student. But on account of persecution because of his views he moved to Vienna after a year, where he won his diploma in 1868. Immediately he returned to Budapest where he began his practice, and most of his supporters followed him there.

Up to 1871 he worked unceasingly on his discovery, and then he saw that the time had come to publish his results. He was requested to give a lecture on his eye-diagnosis to the Hungarian Homoeopathic Society. The lecture was begun, but never finished, for the opponents to his views had disturbed his address in such a manner that Peczely broke it off and declined to go on. After this occurrence he founded a magazine entitled "Iris," in which he placed before the public his researches in the Hungarian and German languages. In the year 1880 the first edition of "Eye-Diagnosis" in Hungarian and German appeared. From then on the interest in Peczely's discovery grew all over the world. He was visited by the most distinguished homoeopathic doctors, such as Stiegele of Stuttgart, Grubermann of St. Gallen, Schlegel of Tuebingen, and Fischer, Physician-in-Ordinary to the Queen of Prussia.

The Homoeopathic Monthly, during the year 1886, contained detailed accounts of his life, eye-diagnosis and his theory. In 1887 Stiegele defended eye-diagnosis against Dr. Sick. Dr. Albert Miller, of San Francisco, was in correspondence with Peczely in 1893, and wished to bring out an English edition of eye-diagnosis. Professor Marques wanted to take the translation in hand, but as he had to move to Honolulu (after the annexation of the Hawaii Islands) in order to save his estates, the above effort fell through. Marques fought for the recognition of eye-diagnosis in the "Mercury." In 1896 Peczely was invited to go to America in order to give lectures to the Homoeopathic Clinics in Philadelphia. He would, however, not undertake this long journey.

In 1881 Dr. Peczely turned his interest to more important matters. Through his discovery in the iris of the mark of bi-sexuality he worked on his great conception of bi-sexuality, the origin of the world, and finally the marvellous laws of procreation, in which he shows the way to eugenics and artificial control in regard to number and sex of the offspring. The public at this time knew of these discoveries just as little as it does to-day. The professional and lay press of Budapest, Vienna, Stuttgart, Berlin,

Bremen, Karlsruhe, Leipzig, Munich, Breslau, Madrid, New York was full of the name of Peczely, particularly in the year 1887, but he is mentioned only as the discoverer of eye-diagnosis.

IRIS PIGMENTATION

The literal meaning of the word "Iris" is a coloured halo or rainbow circle, and so it is used to denote the coloured circular membrane placed between the cornea, the transparent anterior portion (or forefront) of the eye, and the lens, which is a biconvex body (also transparent) lying in a capsule further back behind the pupil—the aperture in the centre of the iris for the passage of light to the light-sensitive nervous back portion of the eye, called the retina.

The coloured iris is a muscular device which is able to relax or contract so as to control the amount of light that enters the eye, like the shutter of a camera. It is the front surface of the iris that may be of different colours or shadings of colour in different individuals, such as blue, brown, grey or green, depending on the amount and distribution of the pigment cells. This colouring is determined largely by heredity.

It is now known, however, that abnormal pigmentation of the iris occurs as a result of nutritional deficiencies which cause serious disturbances of the normal chemistry of the body. This new discovery surely calls for further observations and study, as painstaking as those of Dr. von Peczely.

CHAPTER 17

UNEASY WAKEFULNESS

THERE are probably few of us who have not experienced an uneasy wakefulness at nights after a short time in bed. The brain may not be unduly active, but an uncomfortable warmth is generated with a fullness in the head, and we seek ease by twisting and turning, which produces further stimulation and an increasing warmth.

This state may also arise after waking from an hour or so's disturbed sleep; instead of enjoying a comforting warmth we suffer from a disagreeable heat and head congestion. We try to woo sleep, but all in vain.

A possible explanation for this state of affairs has been suggested by Baron von Reichenbach. He maintains that what he calls an "odic" force permeates, and emanates from, everything in the universe, including every human being, and that where certain physiological conditions are present too much odic force may be generated and may accumulate in the bed. It is this, he claims, that causes uneasiness and objectionable warmth.

The obvious remedy is to get out of bed—overcoming any natural disinclination—and to throw back the bedclothes to allow the accumulated odic force to escape more speedily by a thorough "airing" of the bed. While this is being done, Baron von Reichenbach advises us to don a dressing-gown and stroll around the bedroom, a practice which not only airs the body and cools it, but also helps to break the vicious circle of thoughts. On returning to bed, which will feel delightfully fresh and cool after its discharge of surplus odic energy, the feeling of discomfort will have gone and sleep will come quickly.

Whether Baron von Reichenbach's theory of the accumulation of odic force is correct or not matters little to the sufferers from uneasy wakefulness—*if it works*. The writer has found that it does—better in some individuals than in others, like most things, but it seems to bring some relief to all.

There is another practical aid to sleep which will stop the brain from going "round and round" in those persons who are unable to leave their worries downstairs when they go to bed.

After settling oneself in bed start going over the events of the day *backwards*. Many who have tried this method have, to the writer's knowledge, fallen asleep before even reaching so far as mid-day in their thoughts. But whether one falls asleep or not during the process, it is a most rewarding practice, as things that appeared as problems and difficulties during the day seem to become sorted out and clarified. The practice also improves the memory, for memory has to be exercised as we travel backwards in thought. It also prevents thoughts from chasing themselves in circles until one feels that there is no way out, whereas by reversing our thoughts in chronological order, so to speak, we embark upon a road that is *straight;* usually, long before we reach the end —i.e., the beginning of the day—we unknowingly take a branch road and enter the realm of sweet slumber.

Anyone who, having seen a horror film, full of dreadful situations and ugly incidents, has then seen the same film run through backwards, will have experienced a remarkable sense of relief, the degree of which will be in accordance with his mental and emotional make-up. His mind is brought into a state of equilibrium, as it were. The *"facts"* depicted on the screen have not changed, but when they are viewed in their reverse order they effect a kind of neutralisation of the thoughts and emotions that were generated by the film in the first place. There is a great sense of relief as a murdered hero is seen to come to life again, and nervous and emotional tensions disappear as if by magic.

Viewing a film backwards bears some relationship to the process of retracing, in thought, the events and mental activities which occurred immediately before getting into bed and following them back until the morning's activities are reached—if one can get that far before sleep intervenes, brought about by the freeing of the body and mind from tensions that have been accumulated during the day.

The exercise is of immense value, and well worth a trial, but it must be practised conscientiously until the habit is established. The writer found it most useful in his college days, especially during examinations, since it impressed facts upon the mind and this improves the memory.

It is an excellent method of relieving undue tensions, which are always what might be termed "one-sided." It is like putting a weight in one dish of a scale to balance the weight in the other dish. It establishes equilibrium, which is, fortunately, never stable in actual living. Life would be dull indeed if it were possible to be *always* in a state of perfect balance; nevertheless, it is grand to be able to command it when and where it is needed most.

CHAPTER 18

RHEUMATIC PAINS AND FEATHER BEDS AND PILLOWS

SOME time ago I read in a German medical journal what a Dr. W. Schotten of Berlin had to say about feather beds and pillows in regard to rheumatic pains. I now pass on this information here for the benefit of the countless sufferers from this crippling complaint.

It is a known fact that rheumatic sufferers often experience an increase of pain when they are lying in a feather bed. It has frequently been observed that the pain increased with long lying and that it became almost unbearable when the patient became really warm.

Now one is reminded that warmth in general is really a tried remedy for rheumatism and neuralgic pains, and on applying warmth-giving woollen coverings an appreciable alleviation of the pain is nearly always brought about to some extent.

When in bed with an eiderdown cover, however, we experience otherwise by feeling more pain on becoming warm than is the case with other warm coverings; this can surely justify the assumption that the feathers are the responsible factors for the increase of discomfort.

This question was followed up and the following was ascertained:

When feathers are lightly rubbed together, either with the fingers or with each other, it can be shown that they very quickly become electrically charged. Feathers that have been rubbed against each other have been placed close to a sensitive electroscope, and it could be observed that the needle of the electrical instrument always deviated, an infallible proof that the feathers, after being rubbed, had become electrified.

The electroscope was approached with a pillow that had been slept upon. The needle at once began to oscillate violently. Thus it was clear that the whole of this pillow was pretty strongly charged with electricity.

If one keeps in mind that many sufferers from rheumatism and neuralgia experience more or less severe pain as soon as the atmosphere is charged with electricity, such as is the case before or during a thunderstorm, then we shall understand that the electrical charge surrounding the sufferer plays a decided role in the increase of pain in persons afflicted with rheumatism and neuralgia.

Now, in a feather bed exactly the same thing takes place. Through the body warmth the very thin water-film, i.e., the natural moisture with which, in the normal way, all things are covered, becomes evaporated. That is the reason why one feels coolness and even a slight chilliness immediately after getting into bed. After a short while the body makes less movements and so loses that feeling of coldness to the same degree that the moisture evaporates, which evaporation takes place itself in a heated bedroom. One can check up on this with the aid of a hygrometer. Dry objects charge themselves considerably easier than moist ones.

As regards the bed feathers the matter is as follows:

If the bed is thoroughly aired and remains uncovered for a long time during the day, then its electrical charge will gradually equalise itself with that of the room. The bed absorbs, during the same period, small amounts of moisture from the atmosphere.

When the bed is in use the reverse process takes place, i.e., the bed loses the small amount of moisture, and then an electrical charge of the bed feathers takes place, brought about by bodily warmth and movement, which are transferred to the feathers.

Now, in the degree that the electrically charged feathers increasingly remove electricity from the room and from the sufferer, so must the rheumatic and neuralgic pain increase, becoming severe and, in some cases, finally unbearable.

As not all natural and artificial materials behave exactly in the same way as birds' feathers, so it is now easier to understand why sufferers from rheumatism and neuralgia, who sleep with cotton and woollen coverings are better bedded—at least so far as their pain is concerned—than those who sleep in feather beds and those who rest their heads on feather pillows.

Feather beds have gone more or less out of fashion in Great Britain, but this is not the case with feather pillows, and those patients of mine who have followed my advice by substituting pillows filled with chaff or some other non-feathery substance, have reported that their rheumatic head and neck pains had cleared up or at least had been considerably relieved, and this without any other treatment.

We must not forget, however, that we in this country still use eiderdowns on our beds, which, by the way, are much thinner than the huge plumeau coverings on the German beds. Rheumatic sufferers should discard them.

CHAPTER 19

"EATING CAN BE A DANGEROUS HABIT"
The Musings of a German Dietist

I AM NEVER going to eat again. Eating is unhealthy; it is dangerous. All foods that do me good, harm me. So science maintains.

Take sugar, for instance: it becomes quickly converted into energy. Tests have shown that after athletes have partaken of a meal containing sugar they accomplish more. But a considerable intake of carbohydrates causes decay of teeth. Doctors state that we would be less prone to tooth decay if we consumed less sugar-containing foods.

I must therefore exclude sugar. But stop a bit! Too little sugar in the blood-stream can make me irritable, even to the extent of my committing a crime. It has been found that in the case of robbers and murderers there was too little sugar in the blood.

Therefore, now and again, I must eat a piece of sugar in order to quieten the criminal urge within me. But then, how can I starve the cancer cells that my body may be harbouring? They seem to develop especially well in a blood having a high sugar content. And how shall I prevent having to carry about with me superfluous fat by putting on weight if I have a heart attack and need sugar?

You can understand that I am somewhat nonplussed.

Take spinach now. It may not produce huge muscles, but it contains much iron and calcium and is therefore wholesome, and that is why children should eat it.

But the university professors say that only about a fifth of the iron in spinach is utilised in the body. What is still worse, spinach contains a noxious substance, oxalic acid, which not only binds the calcium in the spinach, but also steals the calcium from other foods that I eat. I am robbed!

I always felt that I did something very special for my health when I nibbled a carrot. It made me feel particularly virtuous. I had learned that carrots contained carotene which the body converted into the coveted vitamin A.

But the latest researches show that the body converts only about a sixth of the quantity it was formerly thought to utilize. If I am to get as much vitamin A as I always thought I should, then I must eat carrots from morning to night, like a rabbit.

With this realization that the vegetable diet does not contain that which has always previously been promised, I turned to animal products—e.g., eggs. Eggs look so nice, don't they? They are a nourishing food, too. Or are they?

Raw white of egg is one of the most indigestible proteins, so states an authorative chemist of the Rockefeller Institute for Medical Research. Of what use is it then to me, when other specialists assert that the protein content in the white exceeds that of the yolk! On the other hand, the cholesterol in the yolk could contribute to the early hardening of my arteries.

Perhaps a cup of coffee would do me good, to clear my head somewhat. It cannot be harmful. But—stop—reverse—no coffee. Coffee can bring about the formation of gastric tumours. This has been proved on both rats and humans. Coffee can also make me restless. But there is a way out. It has also been proved that a little sugar in the coffee exercises a contrary effect. But then I am back to sugar again (see above). In my perplexity I must get hold of some sweetening stuff. But a Hungarian scientist declares that saccharine impairs my precious anti-criminal blood-sugar. Obviously the sweet tooth for saccharine leads the body astray, as it believes that it is getting a supply of the real thing—sugar.

Is there need to wonder, then, that I have decided to live on nothing but bread and water. But only until I have gone more closely into the bread question. I mean, of course, white bread, as tests with mice fed on white bread have shown that they were more capable of resistance to inflammation of the lungs than when fed on wholewheat bread. But white bread is much poorer in health-promoting fats, proteins, and vitamins than the wholewheat. Even when one enriches it with these useful substances it is still no substitute. Besides, the white flour might be bleached with a chlorine compound which brings about convulsions in dogs and could have an influence upon my body in the direction which leads to drunkenness.

There remains for me only the water. Pure water is, if not particularly nutritious, at least a healthful drink. Or is it?

Yes, it is unfortunately thus. Absolutely pure water does not contain the minerals so essential for my body. When I am tired and thirsty and gulp down clear, cold water, this can lead to cramps. If I overdo it the excess water can bring about a mental condition worse than *delirium tremens*.

You will now begin to understand why I have made up my mind to give up eating and drinking, which to the ignorant, appears such a pleasant occupation.

You will likewise appreciate that when someone advises me to eat yeast on account of the vitamin B, I know in advance that somebody else will declare to me that the living yeast cells not only hold on firmly to their own vitamin, but most likely also take the vitamin from my stomach.

So far have I got, then, with my "nutrition," without eating and drinking. But at least I have the certainty of having eliminated everything detrimental to my health. But one moment, please. Perhaps I was too hasty. Perhaps I have read only superficially what the scientists had to say. Perhaps I have not troubled myself to grasp their meaning and have held only to the words. Words are dangerous things. It can easily happen that one can read more into them than is intended.

As gradually, the suspicion arises in me that this decision in regard to my "nutrition" without eating and drinking has a snag in it I decide to reconsider it.

I commence with the yeast. It is quite correct; fresh yeast *does* destroy vitamins—but not so dry yeast. So I could take this. And water is not such an evil after all. If I *will* have it absolutely pure, I can obtain the mineral from other sources. And when I am over-tired I can dissolve a pinch of salt in the water; then I do not get any cramps. And with the exercise of some will-power I shall avoid drinking water by the bucketful.

Neither is bread such an evil when one considers the matter more closely. I can enrich the white bread by supplementing it with other foods. It is not proved that flour which has been bleached by trichlornitrogen has ever done anybody any harm. To be sure, sensitive dogs feeding almost exclusively upon such flour do develop convulsions; but no detrimental effects were evident in a proportion of 1 : 3. But what is of more importance is that this bleaching procedure is now no longer used in the mills.

Wholewheat bread is also in order. It has never made anyone prone to inflammation of the lungs.

I should like to revert to coffee. I have never got tumours from drinking it. Obviously I must belong to the ninety per cent who are immune to its bad influence. It seemingly produces them only in a very small proportion of supersensitives. I certainly do not worry myself that coffee can make me nervous. I believe that, in any case, it is to a great extent imagination. People have been given caffeine-free coffee and they could not sleep. Others were given caffeine-free coffee and they have slept like little babes.

Raw white of egg may be protein difficult to digest, while proteins generally are easily digestible. Anyway, I cook my egg. The theory that the cholestrol in the yolk contributes to the harden-ing or blocking of the arteries is, after all, nothing but a theory. At all events I do not eat one egg less on that score.

I obtain some vitamin A when I eat carrots, and even more from liver and butter. In any case carrots are cheaper. And the oxalic acid in a portion of spinach is no reason for cutting it out from an otherwise good and varied menu.

Now, so far as white sugar is concerned—a pure carbohydrate

86

—it contains neither vitamins nor proteins, mineral salts nor fats. So far as I am concerned, the individual might be right in that there is a connection between excess sugar consumption and tooth decay. But a *little* carbohydrate cannot do much harm when I can silence my conscience by cleaning my teeth afterwards. Anyway, I no longer intend to suck a sweet merely because of the danger that a lack of sugar will irritate my nerves. I have myself sufficiently well in hand not to commit crimes through a lack of sugar. Sweet-eating on the sly I leave to would-be homicides.

I remember that experiments were made in factories. Tit-bits were given to the workers between meals. It is alleged that the production was increased. But perhaps the break had more to do with this than the snack. Recent tests on the effects of refreshments for furthering output have, at all events, yielded no result.

Naturally I would not refuse a piece of chocolate if I felt weak in the middle of a tennis tournament, or if I required extra strength when climbing a mountain. And if I should be adrift on a raft in the middle of the ocean I should be grateful if there were some grape sugar handy. I have read that, through some kind of trick of chemistry, grape sugar will somewhat reduce my desire for water.

In a word, I shall return to the approved balance diet and will alter nothing of importance. I shall also take to heart the words of one of our greatest physiologists who stated that nutrition fit for humans is healthful nutrition for man, woman and child. Only a very few individuals are exceptions in a particular way in that they react abnormally to certain foods—e.g., by a skin eruption after enjoying some strawberries.

Further, the physiologist sees a safety factor as regards a correct diet in that one can include in the menu the animal kingdom as well as the vegetable.

Yes, at the start this scheme of not eating and drinking appeared to me just fine, but now I have come to my senses.

CHAPTER 20

THE "WHY" AND "WHEREFORE" OF MASTICATION

MOST people appreciate that thorough mastication of their food is desirable in the interests of health—that it is good for the teeth and that it helps the digestive processes—but very few appear to know why, and, 'in everyday life the act of mastication receives little or no consideration.

The physiology of digestion has often been dealt with, so in this chapter the subject of mastication will be approached from a somewhat different angle.

Look at a cube—say a cube of sugar. It has six surfaces. If we cut through the three dimensions of the cube we shall have eight smaller cubes each of which will have six surfaces—48 surfaces in all (8 cubes by 6 surfaces). Now, let us divide each of these eight cubes into eight still smaller ones. The result is 64 cubes, each with six surfaces, making a total of 384 surfaces. If each of these 64 very small cubes could be divided further into eight cubelets, we should have 512 cubelets, with no less than 3,072 surfaces. If the process of sub-division were continued, the number of exposed surfaces would increase until the original cube of sugar, which had only six surfaces, was reduced to the granulated state, with many thousands of open surfaces. Nevertheless, **the volume of sugar remains exactly the same as that of the original large cube.**

Now, let us see what all this has to do with mastication.

Put the whole cube of sugar into your mouth, but do not crush it with your teeth. The saliva can reach only six surfaces, and so the sugar will take a long time to dissolve completely. But if the same cube is crushed (or masticated), then the saliva may attack simultaneously the many hundreds of surfaces that have been exposed to its penetrating action.

Crushing sugar with the teeth—especially hard, boiled sweets, is certainly not to be encouraged, nor is it necessary, because the mere act of sucking will, in due time, dissolve it.

The example of the sugar does, however, illustrate why it is of the utmost importance to create, through chewing, as many surfaces as possible, so that the saliva, and eventually the gastric juices, can act upon the tiny particles of solid food more quickly and easily than if large chunks of food had to be dealt with.

In passing, it may be mentioned that starches and ordinary sugars are, or should be, largely predigested in the mouth by the saliva. The more we chew, therefore, the better can the saliva do its work before the food is swallowed. Protein, on the other hand, is digested in the stomach by the action of hydrochloric acid. Why need we bother, then, about chewing meat, for example? Remembering the example of the sugar cube, it will be obvious that by biting into the meat we break it down into particles, and the tinier these particles become under the grinding action of the teeth, the more surfaces will be exposed to the action of the gastric juices when the food reaches the stomach. Also, the mixing of the saliva with the meat particles "liquefies" the bolus, or mass of masticated food, so that swallowing is greatly facilitated; this, of course, applies to all kinds of foods.

If it is difficult to visualise the action of the juices upon the protein in the stomach itself, the following simple, if somewhat crude, experiment will illustrate the process.

Place a two inch cube of meat into a glass jar containing hydrochloric acid. Mince up another two inch cube of the same meat and put it into another glass jar, also containing hydrochloric acid. The quantity of protein is the same in both jars, but it is clear which portion will be "digested" more easily and in the shorter time. In the first case the acid will have to work its way through the mass of compact meat, whereas in the second the minute particles offer less "resistance" to attack by the acid because of the vast number of surfaces exposed to its action.

Now, let us see how the act of mastication affects the salivary glands, teeth, gums, and tonsils.

On each side of the face there are three glands, making six in all. (These are the glands that become affected in mumps). Their job is to secrete what we know as saliva, which, as has already been mentioned, acts upon the starches and sugars of our food.

Some people complain that they cannot eat unless they drink at the same time, because the mouth is too dry. This dryness is brought about over the years because, as a result of insufficient mastication, the salivary glands are not given the necessary stimulus to secrete. If such people, instead of drinking with their meals, would persevere with chewing until the food becomes almost a fluid, the salivary glands would soon become fully active once more and would produce a copious flow of saliva. Furthermore, a keener taste would develop, thus affording a greater enjoyment of every morsel of food.

Teeth and gums need exercise. This results not only in strengthened jaw muscles, but in an increased circulation of the blood to the teeth, gums, and facial muscles. A better drainage of the tonsils is also effected, and there may even be a lessening of some types of noises in the ear and an improvement of catarrhal deafness.

Deep down in his nature, modern man is no less aggressive than his primitive brothers. The aggressive instinct is natural, because it is an instinct, and in a civilised community it may be turned to very good account. The "go-getters," and those who accomplish and construct things in life, evidence the aggressive instinct, sometimes very forcefully, in specialised ways, but unfortunately such people are usually hurried eaters, especially those who are unpleasantly aggressive in their behaviour. Gastric and duodenal ulcers, etc., are recognised to-day to be due to excessive worry and consequent nervous tension. One of the best correctives of this condition is concentrated mastication. Also, there is no better means of overcoming chronic constipation, other things being equal, as well as many other ills of the body and the mind.

Those who suffer from repressed and suppressed aggression may find a natural outlet in biting hard on their food. There is a great satisfaction to be derived from getting your teeth into things, both actually and figuratively. So bite ... bite ... bite your food; keep on biting hard with the full consciousness focused upon the act. Not only will you arise from each meal with an easy, satisfied feeling in the body, and experience a clarity of mind, but you will be more or less freed from noxious aggression, especially when things go wrong.

The practice of chewing with concentrated attention requires discipline, to begin with, but with repetition the habit becomes firmly established. Such discipline also strengthens the will.

Impatience and confused, illogical thinking may be effectively lessened by the simple exercise of refraining from putting any further food into the mouth until the preceding supply has been chewed to a pulp.

The disciplinary act of emptying the mouth of food between one bite and the next will make it easier to deal more effectively with many other situations that may arise. Undue mental and physical tensions may be obviated, or at least reduced, by this practice, with the result that fears, too, will be lessened in intensity. The tension is literally transformed into a healthy form of aggression by the act of attacking one's food.

Thorough mastication, then, has far more to it than the mere breaking down of food into tiny particles for easy digestion.

Conscious direction of the act of eating, so that one is fully aware of the process, constitutes an unusual yet natural method of developing quite a few desirable qualities, and is an effective way of releasing, naturally and harmlessly, emotions that might otherwise remain pent-up, to be let loose, perhaps in a flood of anger and even in violence in an unguarded moment.

CHAPTER 21

THE PYONEX TREATMENT

Very many years ago Carl Baunscheidt, a German, was resting his acutely painful rheumatic hand on a table when he received several stings from a number of gnats. These stings created numerous very tiny openings on the skin through which toxic matter was eliminated by the action of the insect venom, with the result that the rheumatism in the hand completely disappeared never to return.

We, in this country, have heard about the use of bee stings and formic acid given in homœopathic doses in the treatment of rheumatism, and this reminds me to quote here a letter which a former patient of mine wrote about his wife to the editor of *Country Life* on the 13th August, 1948, a copy of which he handed to me. Here it is:

"With reference to your recent correspondence as to the efficacy of bee stings for rheumatism. Some years ago my wife who had been suffering from acute rheumatism in both knees for some months, and had a horror of wasps, asked me to remove one from the room before she got up. This I did, as I thought, and shut the window, but a little later, my wife, on opening the window, received a full sting in the thumb from the wasp. She had a very painful arm for most of the day, but on getting up from her chair after tea, she found that her rheumatism had entirely gone, and it did not return ... "

Now, none of us likes to be stung by a bee, wasp or any other insect, much less deliberately so, hence we have to thank Carl Baunscheidt for discovering a method, whereby this eliminative effect can be produced in regulated doses over any length of time that may be indicated by the nature of the disease and condition of the patient, with very little if any appreciable discomfort.

This eliminative treatment, known in Germany as "Baunscheidtismus" after the name of its discoverer Baunscheidt, was given the name of PYONEX (pus expeller) by an English doctor by the name of Rule, M.R.C.S. He wrote a large work on the subject about the end of the last century, and it was from this volume that I made a study of the method and have practised it over the last twenty-five years.

Dr. Rule's life was once despaired of, but it was saved by the application of Baunscheidtismus, of which he knew nothing at the time. After making a most remarkable recovery, when all other treatments had proved to be ineffective, he devoted the rest of his life to the study and practice of the method, and wrote the book mentioned above, in which I became very interested, so much so that I was after as much information on the subject as it was possible to obtain. Happening to possess a good knowledge of the German language my efforts and patience were at long last rewarded after the war in that I was fortunate enough to be able to obtain from Germany the original books by Carl Baunscheidt, the discoverer himself. These indicated, inter alia, the very wide range of diseases that could be successfully treated by this "pus-expelling" therapy, including various forms of paralysis such as Disseminated Sclerosis about which I wrote in my article that was published in the May, 1952, issue of the *Health and Life* magazine.

Now, what is the "modus operandi" of this method of treatment?

Baunscheidt, after his eliminative, curative experience from the many gnat bites on his hand, referred to at the very beginning of this article, thought that if he could find a way to emulate Nature in her eliminative efforts he would be doing a great service to suffering humanity. So he invented an instrument having thirty-three needles, the bases of which are firmly fixed in a round boss of lead. To the bottom of this boss is firmly attached a closely coiled spring about six inches long. This is enclosed in a circular, narrow, elongated case, which looks roughly like a small round ruler, but tapering somewhat. At one end of this "ruler" there is a thin handle protruding, whilst at the other end is the boss with the needles. The cap is removed and the needle end is now pressed on the skin of the part of the body to be treated. The handle is pulled out an inch or so, thus expanding the spring, and it is suddenly released so that the needles, which project a trifle less than an eighth of an inch, penetrate the epidermis. This is just felt by the patient, but it does not hurt. The object of these needles is to create a number of artificial pores, each set of punctures consisting of thirty-three. This procedure corresponds to the tiny openings made in the skin by the bite of the insect. Into these artificially made pores is now brushed a special oil, made up of three different oils, and this is analogous to the substance that is injected by the biting insect.

In some cases the taps of the instrument are followed in a few minutes by prominent macules, the perforations presenting the appearance of a plucked goose. But the usual course is for this appearance to supervene some hours after the application. The macular stage, after a few hours, is followed by the papular. This papular stage lasts also a few hours. The papules are distinctly formed by the pushing up of the epidermis from beneath and will not disappear on pressure by the finger, as in the case of macules.

In about twenty-four hours the papules begin to merge into vesicles, which stage usually lasts twenty-four hours. During this stage the vesicles become filled with a semi-transparent serum, which has a consistency somewhat thicker than that of ordinary serum. The vesicles continue to increase in size and their contents gradually become more opaque, until at the termination of forty-eight hours they merge into pustules. This pustalar stage lasts twenty-four hours. The whole process takes about forty-eight hours from the time the oil is applied until the pustules are formed. The part or parts treated are covered by a layer of cotton wool.

When the morbid element does not exist in large quantities, or when it is not of an irritant nature, the skin which is *between* the sets of perforations may retain its natural appearance throughout the whole period of the treatment, but in severe cases the pustules are not confined to the perforations of the needles, but absolutely cover the whole cutis so completely, that it is not possible to lay the head of a pin on any part without touching a pustule. These pustules are smaller than those at the perforations.

On the fourth or fifth day a second crop of pustules are sometimes thrown out, which are sporadic, and usually not very numerous; they are or may be filled with pus which is a deeper shade in colour.

The oil has the peculiar property of increasing the vitality, which is communicated to any part by the Pyonex Treatment, so that the increased temperature and activity in the circulation combine to attract to the part the exciting cause of the disease, which has been lodging say in a neighbouring joint, or some of the deeper tissues. The exciting cause then becomes eliminated.

Blisters, mustard, poultices and stimulating liniments act in the same manner; *but in a far less degree.* Being applied externally, i.e., on the surface of the skin only, although their use is attended so often by excellent results, yet they are of no avail in stubborn cases. But the stimulating Pyonex oil passes through the artificial pores, into the soft tissues, and is carried by the circulation into their midst, keeping up its vitalising action for three days, instead of only for a few hours, and in this way enables the system to carry out its own process of elimination on such a scale as can be attained by no other means.

It is sufficiently evident that in some affections the expulsive efforts which are made by Nature, are so weak and ineffective, that the quantity of toxic matter expelled makes no material difference to the progress of the disease. A few pustules may be thrown out here and there, which may be taken as signs of the mass of virus, embedded in the deeper tissues, which the unaided powers are wholly incapable of dislodging or expelling.

By the judicious application of the Pyonex Treatment, we have it in our power to remove obstacles, and to furnish such aids as may prove effectual to our obtaining the end in view.

By making artificial pores, we tap the envelope of the epidermis, and provide a suitable exit for all kinds of purulent and morbid products that may be harboured in the system.

By the subcutaneous introduction of the oil, the impaired vitality of the part is overcome; and active circulation is promoted and while on the one hand, the offending impurity is thus reached, and expelled from its lurking place, on the other hand, the natural reproductive powers are resuscitated, and there is set up a process of re-installation of new and healthy tissue.

When the pus is lodged in the deeper tissues, it may be successfully reached and expelled, by repeated applications. The impurity which is nearest to the surface, naturally is the first to reach the new pores, and as the treatment is continued, the deeper tissues are compelled to disgorge, until not a vestige remains behind, and not a pustule can be produced by further application of the Pyonex.

In cases of paralysis, however, notwithstanding this fact, it is necessary to continue the applications, the object being to excite the tissues to a healthy growth and vitality. The spinal column is, of course, the part to which special attention is directed in these cases, but the individual treatment of the limbs which are affected, is necessary in order to obtain more satisfactory results, as they are usually charged with offending elements.

The increased vitality communicated to a part by repeated applications of the Pyonex treatment is evidenced in several ways, among which are the following:

Vascularity: The increase of activity in the vascular system is marked. The arteries and veins which for weeks or years have been shrunk and withered, rapidly increase in calibre, and the resulting new supply of blood to the part similarly affects the cellular tissues, nervous peripherae and capillaries.

Healing Power: The healing power of the whole system, and especially the parts contiguous to the application, is improved. Discharging sores and wounds of long standing begin to show a healthier appearance, and end by closing up. In a case, for example, of fissure of the anal sphincter, which had been discharging for years, it healed in a few weeks, the cure being permanent. In cases of curvature of the spine which are not due to malformation, the muscles increase in volume and tone, and the result of their increased vitality is to pull the column into a straight line; the abnormal curves disappear, and every vertebra resumes its natural position.

Increase in sensation and muscle-tone usually supervenes in a short time when the treatment is given in cases of paralysis and *locomotor ataxia.* The quantity of purulent matter which is expelled in the latter disease is at times beyond anything that one would believe possible; this is after the first two or three applications, after which there is a marked diminution in quantity, as is to be expected.

It was a custom among medical practitioners forty or fifty years ago to make what was called an "issue," in any part of the body, where there was a fixed pain or other symptoms, which could not be relieved by ordinary methods. This was done by cauterising a circular spot on the skin about the size of a shilling; the centre of this spot was cauterised to a sufficient depth to retain a pea, which was secured in its position by adhesive plaster. By this plan the part was precluded from healing and continuous suppuration was maintained. An outlet was thus established by which the morbid element which caused the pain was expelled from the system.

The action of the Pyonex treatment is similar to that of an "issue." Its action is not, however, confined to a small spot, as in the case of the "issue," but may, in case of need, be extended over the whole of the chest, abdomen and back, so that whatever morbid elements may have lodged in any part of the system, an exit is provided in their immediate proximity, by which they may be expelled.

The "issue," mentioned above, which was kept open by means of a pea, was maintained in this state as a rule for weeks, in order to accomplish the desired end. The exit being small and isolated, and the natural forces being unaided, the excreting of the morbid matter was necessarily slow. But in the case of the Pyonex treatment, the expulsion of blood poisons, and of morbid and foreign elements, is greatly accelerated, not only because of the four or five thousand exits that are provided by the artificial pores made by the needles, but also by the absorption into the tissues and circulation of the stimulating oil, which conveys to the part new life and vigour.

To every point where the inherent healing power has been reduced to a low ebb by the presence of so much impurity, which must naturally be attended to by a sound dietetic régime, the inrush of the oil brings the stimulus that is needed. The new volume and rapidity of the current of the blood are such, that the barriers which are met with in the semi-consolidated tissues are soon broken down and dissipated. By the accomplishment of this, the disease toxins which were so long deposited in the affected parts are dislodged, and expelled through the artificial pores; the surrounding tissues, no longer burdened by morbid productions, soon resume a healthy tone, and the natural forces have again a free hand in building up a healthy system.

It will be seen therefore that the main beneficial and curative effect of the Pyonex depends upon the expulsion of morbific matter from the system. Hence the main object to be kept in view during treatment is to establish and maintain the expulsive action at its most effective point. That is why this form of therapy is so successful in the treatment of such diseases as bronchitis, asthma, pneumonia, pleurisy and indeed in some types of cases of the intractible disease, arthritis. It is very effective too in skin diseases and even in the treatment of that much-talked-of complaint these days known as "slipped disc," and in support of this I submit a report of a case of Herniated Disc which was published in *The British Nauropathic Association News,* July-August, 1950, issue:

"Male aged thirty-six. In 1935 patient fell off a ladder on to his back. Very acute pain resulted; could not bend in any direction. Confined to bed for six weeks. Later was X-rayed; an adjustment was made to the lumbar spine under an anaesthetic by a manipulative surgeon at a hospital. Then a course of lumbar injections was followed by massage and radiant heat. Still more pain, which was intensied after the manipulation by the surgeon. Three years ago patient was put into a plaster jacket. Still no relief. Constant headaches. Sleeping tablets had to be taken. Two years ago X-rayed again. Two surgeons independently diagnosed herniated disc and ordered operation. Patient, however, refused, but continued to suffer greatly and was unable to attend his work. Osteopathic treatment was commenced by me on 6th September, 1949, but this was dropped after three treatments in favour of the Pyonex treatment only, owing to the very congested state in the lumbar spine area. This treatment caused a drainage through the skin of purulent matter. Relief was experienced from the first Pyonev treatment and after only ten such weekly treatments, the whole condition cleared up. The transformation in the patient was truly amazing, as well it might be after a liberation from great and handicapping pain from which the patient had suffered since 1935. This 'decongesting' treatment has been used in many such cases with equal success."

The editor of the *B.N.A. News,* Mr. Milton Powell, M.B.N.A., had this comment to make at the time:

"This case would seem to confirm the view that disc trouble may not always be due to direct pressure from the displaced cartilage, but rather from the exudative products induced by the original trauma."

Although over twenty-five years have now elapsed since I was lent Dr. Rule's textbook on the Pyonex treatment, I can clearly remember that this doctor postulated that disease was due to the accumulation of morbific matter in the body, and since the organism being overloaded with toxins was unable satisfactorily to eliminate them through the usual channels of bowels, kidneys, skin and lungs some means had to be used whereby this elimination could be accomplished as quickly as the nature of the case would allow. All this is very sound so far as it goes and such a means he found in the PYONEX. But the point I wish to make here is that Dr. Rule does not appear to have made any enquiry into the actual CAUSE of this accumulation of morbid matter, and whilst I can unhesitatingly testify to the efficacy of the Pyonex therapy, yet I cannot conclude this article without stressing the absolute necessity for sufferers to adopt the means whereby a further accumulation of toxins can be *PREVENTED* after they have been expelled, so that the PYONEX or any other form of eliminative treatment in the future may become unnecessary.

CHAPTER 22

STAMMERING AND ITS CURE

I⊤ ɪs the earnest hope of the writer that the two home treatments given herein for dealing with that most distressing complaint of stammering will prove as effective as it has been with his own patients. It is hoped too, that the information will be useful to all those concerned with stammerers viz: parents, teachers and others who are in charge of children.

This chapter is written as much for adults who stammer, as it is for children who are afflicted with this kind of speech impediment, but be it noted, I am confining my observations solely to that speech defect known as stammering or stuttering, which is not occasioned by any anatomical or structural abnormality of the organs of speech. It is thus curable without having recourse to surgical measures.

There is an essential difference between a stammer and a stutter, and this I maintain in spite of the synonymy of the two words as given in a dictionary. Stuttering is a convulsive repitition, whereas stammering is a blocking of speech.

It used to be thought that on training left-handed children to be right-handed there was a danger of their becoming stammerers or stutterers. This appears now to be an old wives' tale. Where the danger can lie, however, is in using FORCE in trying to effect the change over. The child can be aware of an element of cruelty, and if he be a sensitive nature, an inhibition can be induced resulting eventually in a stammer.

The medical examination having established the integrity of the speech organs themselves, the cause of the trouble must be sought for elsewhere. Experience teaches that the defect can be due and traced to inhibitions brought about maybe by some shock or fright, or indeed by sustained mental tensions as the result of anxiety; but parents and others must not confuse—which they are very apt to do—the non-fluency of speech in children with stammering. Parents and teachers are then prone constantly to reprove the child in severe tones for his hesitancies. This in turn, has the effect of making him self-conscious of the manner in which he speaks, and, as a result of this self-centring he becomes nervous. Hence through admonitions shot at him from time to time to speak "properly" a true, honest-to-goodness stammer develops out of what was originally nothing but an ordinary and very common hesitancy, which is more in evidence in some children than in others. This hesitancy in speech is certainly not confined merely to children, for are not all adults more or less subject to this peculiarity of being non-fluent in their daily conversational intercourse with their fellow beings? Just note how various types of people respond with the spoken word when being interviewed on television or radio. Notice too the varied and many hesitancies that manifest themselves in speeches made through these mediums, not to say anything about the non-fluency of even every day small 'talk of ordinary folk. Therefore, the er—ers' and other meaningless sounds must not be confused with a predominant speech defect such as true stammering. Rather are they, more often than not, unconscious devices used in order to gain time when one is at a loss for words appropriate to the occasion or subject-matter in hand. These sounds serve to fill in a blank, what would otherwise be felt as an embarrassing silence. This lack of facility to command an uninterrupted flow of words can be attributed to a variety of reasons, perhaps the chief of which is undue nervousness whilst facing an audience, or it can be due to nervous tensions when dealing with difficult people or with people in difficult situations. There must indeed be very few of us who can get on to our hind legs to deliver a fluent after-dinner speech, or say anything before a television microphone without shaking at the knees, or experiencing an "all-gone" feeling in that region, or without being unpleasantly aware of "butterflies" in the tummy. Some find the greatest difficulty even to put questions at a public meeting. But hypnotherapy would soon free most of these cases from their nervous tensions and consequent nervousness.

There is a number of factors involved in the development of speech. No infant is capable of articulating words, but in every newly born babe the speech potential is present. It is situated in a region of the brain known as Broca's area, which, curiously enough is located only on the left side of the brain in right-handed persons. Now, whether the child will eventually speak English, French, German, Chinese or any of the many hundreds of different languages extant and fluently at that with good pronounciation, enunication, modulation, intonation will naturally depend upon his geographical and educational environment, and also upon his physique and general state of health.

Language, therefore, is an acquired art, the beginnings of which are automatically learnt in early childhood, progress in an increase of vocabulary being made right through to adulthood and then on and on through life consistent with one's educational background and literary tastes, aptitudes, general development and mental make-up.

Stammering or stuttering is due to an interference to the easy flow of words forming sentences, and this interference is due mostly to psychological causes, which, in turn, create physiological disturbances, especially affecting the rhythmic breathing, the lips and tongue, so that the organs of speech are unable to perform their normal function. Those who are afflicted with this distressing habit of stammering usually seek the services of a teacher specialising in speech training. Whilst I am all in favour of voice production, which entails training in regulated breathing, so essential to beauty of speech, and also training in the correct use of the tongue and lips, which training most people sadly need, it leaves the basic cause of the stammer untouched.

Everyone of us would derive great benefit, in more ways than one, by undergoing a course of instruction in the art of speaking at the hands of a competent teacher of elocution, but the stammerer requires something more. He does not need to be TAUGHT speech as such, for that faculty is present at birth and has developed already in his early life in the otherwise normal individual. What IS required, however, is the removal of the inhibiting factor or factors that prevent him from exercising this faculty freely.

As already stated, in most cases there is nothing wrong with the actual speech apparatus itself, but rather with its *manner* of use.

It is common knowledge that the stammerer can read aloud and even recite fluently when alone, and still more easily can he sing words of a song. He can do all this in public too with far more comfort than if he has to speak, for the rhythm and the words, being ready made, keep him on the rails as it were, over which they travel easily. This frees him from undue strain. There are even occasions when in company he loses himself completely in what he is saying, so that there is not a trace of his impediment. This proves the point that the sufferer from this kind of speech defect CAN speak well on the rare occasions, when conditions for him are just right, e.g. when attention is drawn from himself.

I repeat that it is not training in speech as such that is called for by getting the stammerer to utter phrases like "how now brown cow" or "the sea cease-eth but it suffice-eth us," which latter even a good speaker would find it difficult to enunciate distinctly without some practice—but that the cause of the impediment should be sought in the Psyche and brought into the light of consciousness by hypnotherapy which embraces hypnoanalysis.

I shall now give three methods of treating stammering or stuttering, two of which can be undertaken in one's own home, and the third in the consulting room of a hypnotherapist.

1. THE FORCED STAMMER

The stammerer is instructed deliberately to produce an exaggerated stammer and to indulge in the practice of forcing the stammer in the privacy of his own room, or at any opportune place and time. He must put all the effort he can into producing the worst possible stammer of which he is capable, and to sustain the effort in talking against all the resistance he can command. He will soon find this exercise to be such a strenous business that he will be more than glad to revert to ordinary speech, which he will now feel to be so easy by comparison because of the release from the consciously imposed tension in keeping up an enforced stammer. This release can be so great that there is now little or no stammer at all on resuming ordinary speech in the company of other people. Obviously this intentional forced stammer must be practised over and over again.

Now, although this method does not directly reach the basic cause, it can bring about in the course of time, such an improvement in fluent speech that the original cause of the stammer becomes inoperative in producing it; it loses its power.

This method was devised by a Dr. Knight Dunbar, but the principle was known and used by Demosthenes 350 years B.C. He was afflicted with a very severe stammer, but he was determined to get the better of it, and to this end he put pebbles into his mouth in order to INCREASE HIS IMPEDIMENT and to FORCE himself by almost superhuman efforts to overcome his speech defect. And he succeeded too, in that he became the greatest orator of ancient Greece. Stammerers go ye and do likewise!

We have the same principle at work in the training of patients to relax. They are told to tense to the utmost limit their arms their legs and later the whole of the body, and to keep up this tensing business for as long as possible. At last they have to give in through strain-fatigue, whereupon they will experience what relaxation really feels like after the severe self-induced tensions which have been superimposed upon those unconsciously present. It is just this extra forced tension, especially of the speech organs that the stammerer deliberately makes, that causes him to be so aware of his ease when he relinquishes the strain; hence his speech is facilitated, and as he progresses, so his confidence increases and his pleasure in conversational intercourse is established.

2. THE SLEEP METHOD

Although this method appears to be but little known, it is by no means new. It is, however, only comparatively recently that it has been scientifically investigated and experiments made on sleeping persons especially in the United States of America with excellent results.

The procedure requires the services of either parent or a liked parent-substitute in the case of a child. It can be very effectively used for all kinds of improvement purposes, e.g. educative, the removal of any bad habit and unreasonable fears evoking interest in home and school work, enhancing the ability to pass examinations without anxiety, improving the health and accomplishments such as music, art, sports, athletics, and for imparting instruction generally (I refer readers to my book *"Curative Hypnosis—Suggestion and Meditative Relaxation."*)*

The parent is to sit at the bedside of the sleeping child. He is to place his hand lightly on the forehead and then gently stroke it. This has the effect of establishing a sympathic rapport between the parent and child. This is akin to the hypnotic state so that the parent is in "contact" with or can reach the unconscious mind of the child. Appropriate suggestions can now be given to the sleeper, the child being assured that mummy (or daddy) is with him, and that he is to continue to sleep. The suggestions of what the child is to be improved in or freed from had better be prepared and written down beforehand, so that there is an easy flow of words, these suggestions must be repeated over and over again in a subdued voice night after night. Becoming absorbed by the unconscious mind they fulfil themselves in the waking life of the individual, the child being told, whilst still asleep, that he will become fully conscious of the suggestions given and that he can thus enhance their value by using his intelligence and direct them to the best advantage by his own WILL. By this method the WILL can be made stronger and the nervous system strengthened, and emotional states satisfactorily dealt with. I remember reading somewhere that a chimpanzee at the zoo cannot THINK its way out of an EMOTIONAL problem, neither can a human being, he can only be *TRAINED* out if it, and hypnotherapy can accomplish this in the majority of cases.

3 HYPNOTHERAPY

Hypnotherapy in the consulting room is the techique of choice, for it not only follows more or less the same procedure as the sleep method in a more professional way, but in addition it embraces hypnoanalysis which facilitates the tracing and recall of the cause of the trouble. It then brings it to the surface, during which process the actual living over again of the original incident that was responsible for producing the stammer or any other functional trouble, takes place. This "living over" is known in psychotherapeutic circles as an abreaction, and is so effective in dispersing the complaint for all time if it is thoroughly experienced.

The fact must not be lost sight of that unnecessary inhibitions with which the stammerer is afflicted can handicap him in different ways over and above his stammer, throughout his life. These too can be eradicated by hypnotherapy in suitable cases.

Hypnosis is well in the public eye these days, and medically it has made much progress during the last few years. There is no question of imposing the will upon the patient, but rather the

---

* *Published by Thorsons Publishers Limited, 91 St. Martins Lane, London, W.1. Price 7s. 6d. Postage 9d.*

hypnotherapist makes the patient use HIS own Will to cure him. It is the will of the patient to get well. It is the will of the hypnotherapist to get him well. Both wills are thus in harmony and the desired result is the more likely to occur.

The hypnotic state is nothing more or less than *a condition of profound relaxation,* which is brought by employing the CONDITIONING technique as described in my book *"Curative Hypnosis"* already referred to. Relaxation having been induced the obstructions to the innate healing forces of the organism are thus removed and they are aided by powerful curative suggestions. It is the unconscious mind that governs the heart's activity, the circulation, the digestive processes, the glandular secretions, the growth of the hair, of the nails, and so on, to the extent that hindrances to its function will permit. Hypnotic suggestions can exercise a beneficient influence upon this great inner mind, and remove inimical tensions, even reviving the instinct for the selection of health giving foods, as well as those most suitable for slimming in a natural way.

It will no doubt be readily gathered from what is written herein about stammering, that we are not directly concerned with the treatment of the speech defect itself in action, but rather with the discovery and removal of its impedimental CAUSE, of which the stammer is but the EFFECT. There are present inhibitory factors preventing the easy flow of words, but once these are removed, then there are no longer any obstructions to hinder fluent speech.

CHAPTER 23

WHAT IT MEANS TO BE AN ADULT

COME TO think of it, how many of us are really "grown up?" Saint Paul must have recognised that a person, on having reached the age of adulthood, is not necessarily grown up in the sense that he is mentally mature, for paraphrased, did not the great Saint write "When I was a child I did and acted as a child, but when I became an adult I put away childish behaviour and acted as a mature person."

Looking around one, and at ourselves too, one finds indeed very few who conduct themselves as fully matured individuals after having attained the years of adulthood, and this statement will find support in what follows. The subject matter will be dealt with under these headings: OBJECTIVITY-EGOCENTRICITY, TENSION CAPACITY, SUBJECT-OBJECT.

OBJECTIVITY-EGOCENTRICITY:

Let me explain what is meant by "objectivity:" a boy on overhearing his mother saying she would very much like to have a certain gadget made for the kitchen, at once sets about constructing such a gadget. He is greatly interested in the preparations and especially in the work on the thing itself. He undertakes the job with zest.

Now, a young pal is watching him with some envy for he greatly covets the praise that is meted out to the busy lad by some of his parents' friends who see how deftly the youngster uses his hands. The latter, however, is in no way distracted from the work in hand by the pleasing remarks. The other boy can no longer stand hearing this praise, so butts in exclaiming that he too, can make a gadget and a much better one at that, which indeed may be true, and soon proceeds to do so, but—and please note this—from an entirely different motive from that which moved boy number one to make something that his mother would find useful.

The first boy's action is objective, that is; he works objectively for the objective purpose of doing something practical for his mother, whereas the second boy, whilst working somewhat object-ively is doing so for a purely egocentric reason viz: so that he may gain greater praise for HIMSELF begrudging it to his friend.

In writing this the thought has just occured to me that one should never, never praise the CHILD, but what he does, what he accomplishes. His attention will then not be drawn to his own ego, but to the actual WORK done by him, in which he will take more interest and try to excel. He is thus being trained in objectivity, so that he becomes less and less egocentric, which is a centring upon the self.

The awarding of prizes, in schools especially, is really not a very good plan, is it? The prize is the goal not the actual accomplishment which might merit the award. One works in order to gain a prize, the work to be done is merely incidental to that achievement, and not for the objective purpose of eventually being of service to the community.

Children are really trained in egocentricity. How many times a day can be heard: "You NAUGHTY child, you NAUGHTY little thing!" The attention of the child is drawn to ITSELF and not to the wrong committed. It is the THING DONE that is naughty, and it is just THIS the child should be made aware of, OBJECTIVELY observing it. It should also be explained to the child, whenever this may be necessary, WHY it is naughty for him to do such a thing. It is but natural that the child should be egocentric, and the younger he is the more egocentricity does he display, but as he grows older this must become less through training, otherwise he is going to have a very hard time of it in his adult life.

Unfortunately, observation of one's fellow-men reveals that perhaps the majority of them are more egocentric than objective, and although they may appear to act—and indeed do act—objectively, they are all the time doing so for egocentric reasons. Hence it follows that when undertaking anything, we should be quite clear as to our real motives, not sheltering behind any activity that is apparently objective in its aim, when it but serves to advance our own ego or importance.

The main thing is to be absolutely honest with oneself so as to avoid the hypocrisy that is unconsciously wrapped up in the apparent objectivity which, however, is used for egocentric ends. The person who does a thing with his tongue in his cheek is at least honest with HIMSELF.

Objectivity can serve egocentric purposes, but egocentricity can never serve objective aims for the good of the community. What good that might arise is purely incidental, and is not directly due to objective action for the objective purpose of trying to achieve it. For instance, a guest, who is an accomplished pianist, is invited to play at a private party, declares that she cannot play a note this evening. We have met this kind before. Her egocentricity thoroughly enjoys being pressed aloud by her hostess, and then "succumbs" to the popular pressure of the guests present by at last sitting down at the piano. Her rendition of the piece is brilliant, and she revels in the well deserved applause that follows. She certainly behaved objectively in the execution of her art, but does she, in this particular instance, give her performance mainly to bestow pleasure upon her listeners or solely for the purpose of getting the limelight on herself personally, just using the occasion to satisfy her egocentric needs.

Now, of course, we must not enter into any analysis of the MOTIVE of any artist when listening to or seeing his performance. We must give ourselves up to the enjoyment of it. The motive, in such an instance, is of no consequence to us, but it is, or should be, a matter of real concern to the artist himself, for if he be predominantly objective in his exposition with the objective purpose of affording the greatest possible pleasure to his audience, then he himself will derive the greater satisfaction, which in turn, can result in greater achievement.

The word "predominant" has been used advisedly here for the reason no one can possibly be wholly objective in his conduct, neither would it be desirable if it were possible. It is essential and expedient that we should possess some degree of egocentricity. Without a little centring upon oneself one could become neglectful of personal appearances for example, and a state of indifference could arise. A certain amount of pride in one's person and in one's talents and accomplishments is indeed necessary and justifiable, but for the attainment of a fuller, happier and healthier life of all concerned, we must be predominantly objective—otherwise we lack consideration for others.

TENSION CAPACITY

Tension capacity in an individual is the ability to sustain tension, in time, between a need and its satisfaction. This capacity to bear tension until the need can be satisfied, indicates the extent the adult has "grown up." Let me clarify this: the baby is conscious of hunger, and immediately he becomes aware of his need, he cannot wait a second before it is attended to. He yells and keeps on yelling until he is put to his mother's breast or is given the bottle. Here there is no tension capacity at all, and no one does, or can, expect it at that early age. But as the child grows older he learns to wait, and according to his ability at the time and the urgency of his need, he will, more or less, succeed in displaying some patience. Note the "urgency of the need," for the greater it is the more discipline must be exercised to bear the tension. This lack of tension capacity can be seen everywhere.

Come with me now into a crowded restaurant. A middle aged man sits down at our table, and hardly is he seated when he calls the waiter without even first consulting the menu. It so happens that this particular waiter does not include our table in his allocation, and on this being pointed out to the impatient individual, who, let us assume, is not in any hurry, he shows annoyance; but he is unable to contain himself and calls out to another waiter.

When he does come along, after having attended to other earlier patrons, he is "told off" for his dilatoriness, then an order is given for some dish that will take at least ten minutes to prepare according to the menu. In spite of this he unreasonably expects to be served almost without delay, and not being so he seeks out the supervisor, who has to exercise tact, without being unfair to the waiters, when dealing with such refractory people. Now our man, not being in any hurry to take his departure, sips his coffee, lights a cigar and reads his paper.

Many times have I witnessed such impatient behaviour viz: the inability to wait a reasonable time for the need to be satisfied. Here we have the conduct of a very young child, which is normal or natural enough at that stage of development, but quite out of place later in life. Such people have not grown up; they have not become true adults; they are not fully mature mentally.

OBJECT-SUBJECT

"I" in grammar is the "subject," whilst the person referred or spoken to is the "object." This is all right and proper so far as grammar is concerned, but not in our dealings with our fellow-men, as we shall see.

Let us start with a husband and his wife. He correctly feels that he is a subject in his own right. How many times in the day does he use the first personal pronoun "I?" But his wife equally uses it too, and why not; is she not a subject too in her own right? Yet her husband unwittingly treats her as an OBJECT, an object of his love, an object of his support, an object of looking after his needs, and, occasionally, an object of his hatred, an object of this that and the other. But is the wife any the less guilty; does she not too, look upon her husband as an object in more or less the same way? And does she not treat him as such?

Then there are the children. How many of us ever give a thought to the fact that they also are subjects no less than ourselves, each possessing his or her own intelligence and individuality. Yet, are they not treated very much like OBJECTS, objects of love, objects of expense, objects of worry, of annoyance, etc., etc? Indeed they are—to their great detriment. What about the slave market—one of the most outstanding examples of human beings being treated as objects? What about the present-day colour bar in this respect and employers and employees each viewing the other as objects?

How greatly the health and happiness of all of us would improve if only we remembered to treat each other as subjects, notwithstanding our differences, which after all, make us individuals for then tolerance and understanding would be exercised. What vexations, distresses and anxieties and anger, would be spared by recognising that excessive egocentricity can be responsible for these obnoxious emotional states so inimical to our well-being.

Attaining and maintaining health is not just a matter of diet alone. One becomes heartily sick of the word when it is over emphasised—as if diet by ITSELF was the end and be all of one's existence! Of course sensible feeding is of great importance, but without a happy, optimistic disposition it is not of much use, for it is not WHAT one puts into the stomach that matters, but what the tummy is able to make of the food when it is there. So let us try to be predominantly objective in our everyday behaviour, so that our activities may be constructive and uplifting. Let us treat each other as SUBJECTS and not as mere objects, and lastly, but by no means of less importance, let us cultivate mental tension capacity, so that we may learn how to wait with patience in an easy, relaxed state of mind.

For those who are desirous of ridding themselves of undue mental and physical tension, may I recommend them to read the last chapter of my book *"Curative Hypnosis"* on *"Meditative Relaxation."*

CHAPTER 24

THE RESISTING EGO

IT HAS long been known to psychologists, neurologists, and for that matter, other healers as well, that certain types of patients, classified as neurotics, do not—deep down in themselves—wish to get well, incomprehensible as this must appear to the man in the street. This strange and apparently illogical desire can apply equally to those suffering from so-called organic disease, in spite of the fact that the methods of treatment adopted for effecting a cure are by no means rejected by the patient, but—and this is the point—he will accept them only on certain conditions being fulfilled. For example, he will agree to undergo a certain form of treatment, but will raise all kinds of objections to whatever other form of therapy that the practitioner may deem, by his specialised knowledge and experience, to be the more effective. Should the practitioner assert his professional authority by insisting upon his method being carried out, then the patient may outwardly appear to obey, while inwardly revolting all the time. The method is most likely doomed to failure at the very outset.

In this way does the patient guard his beloved ego. In the light of his full consciousness it is obvious to him, as indeed it is to others, that getting well is of immense concern to him, but the preservation of his own ego is of far greater importance, and should recovery signify the "sacrifice" of the ego, then he remains ill, in spite of all his own efforts and those of his physician to restore him to health.

All this is, of course, unconscious. The intelligent, reasonable, conscious self continues its search for health by trying this remedy, then that, by going to this doctor, to that naturopath or osteopath, to this Nature Cure Home and to that Hydro, but we all so well know, deriving little or no benefit from any.

It is evident that he is involved in a vicious circle. There must be some inhibiting factor preventing his complete or partial recovery.

Close observation reveals that if there be any one factor responsible for his ailment, it will be found in the patient's own *egocentricity*, and egocentricity contains innumerable factors in itself. The patient himself is not aware of this, because egocentricity is the outcome of his early training, of his behaviour patterns or style of life originating from infancy. We are all products of our training formulae which result in conditioning us to behave in the way we do, thus these are powerful forces in our lives, and so long as we remain ignorant of them, they are responsible for much unhappiness and ill-health.

Consider this very simple illustration: few of us can tolerate a flat contradition, especially in a heated argument. According to the circumstances, we flare up and defend our point of view in a most unreasonable way, but in reality, what we are defending is our own precious ego. Were it not so, the severe defence would not produce nervous prostration, hysteria, digestive and other bodily disturbances. This constant and blind defence of the ego, irrespective of truth or logic—this continual attempt to "save our face" at any price—MUST and does lead to physical malfunctioning and thus to illness. Then so long as the physician, the family or others can minister to our egocentricity, we get, more or less well. Here is a condition being fulfilled to the satisfaction of the patient. Sufferers want to get cured of their symptoms, but how often are they willing to accept the means in full, whereby that desirable end may be attained? There is always a "BUT." These patients unconsciously fight against clarification, because there is a subtle awareness that, were this to be brought about, it would mean their having to accept the responsibilities of life and facing up to its difficulties.

Now, if the individual's early training formulae are the unconscious factors ruling his life, how can the cure take place? Here are suggested three possible ways:—

1. By the practitioner possessing adequate knowledge of character and of the workings of the human mind, not only causing the patient to become aware of the nature of his training formulae, but also of his goal. He must also be able to make the patient see that the possible attainment of his goal is being accomplished at the expense of so much bodily suffering and mental distress through his, all unknown to him, egocentric behaviour patterns, thus depriving him of full enjoyment of the satisfaction of complete and unfettered achievement.

The practitioner must endeavour to make his patient recognise that the same goal, or a better one, can be attained by objective behaviour for OBJECTIVE purposes. This latter is all-important for the cure. In other words, objective aims must be substituted for egocentric ones.

2. By the treatment not interfering with the egocentric aims of the patient; but this is negative in its results, for it means that the patient is for ever dependent upon his doctor, who unwittingly panders to his patient, and so long as he (the doctor) continues to be the patient's contact person, as the mother, father, sister, brother or wife were in the past, so long will the patient be tied to the physician. When that ceases, the "cure" is undone and the patient goes on his fruitless search for health in the never ending vicious circle.

3. By the patient himself—without any aid—realising the unconscious purpose or goal his ailment is serving, and then being willing to renounce, not necessarily the purpose, but rather the MEANS of attaining it, namely, his egocentricity, which results in his illness.

One can say that many a person feels, and rightly so, but unconsciously, that "being in health" is a very difficult business, while consciously he allows himself to be deluded into fantasying a goal of sham well-being, namely, happiness without any bothersome means to attain it, thus evading all responsibility. The more apparent it becomes, as treatment proceeds, that this way does not lead to that dreamland of happiness, but rather to those very difficulties which go to make up life as a whole, and without which no complete life can be experienced, all the greater resistances does the patient put up against such enlightenment. So long as the patient entertains a false idea of what health really is, he is not sufficiently prepared for a cure. This is the physician's job, but hardly any doctor gives a thought to the overwhelming egocentricity of his patient, SIMPLY BECAUSE HE (THE PHYSICIAN) HIMSELF IS QUITE UNAWARE OF HIS OWN EGOCENTRIC BEHAVIOUR. Here it is a case of "Physician heal thyself!" Life in the kingdom of health must be prepared for by the practitioner and learnt by the patient, just as life in a foreign country, and any treatment that omits this "positive-training" logically increases the resistances of the patient.

The breaking down of resistances can be accomplished by bringing about an improved point-of-view, a clarification, and by making the patient realise that happiness cannot be attained by the way of fantasied conditions surrounding the idea of health; but health for health's sake must be striven for, so that OBJECTIVE purposes may be fulfilled. The GOAL health must become the MEANS to achieve the greater goal of a full, objective life. Secondly, there must be a clear conception of what health really is, namely, a harmonious working of the organism as a whole, both mental and physical. It does not mean a fool's paradise or Utopia without suffering, without difficulties, but work and development and all the responsibility that is part and parcel of a real active life.

It is erroneous to say: "I could perhaps achieve health IF only I had the strength, but life has so dealt with me that I cannot possibly go on." That is just an excuse, which originates from the false notion that ENERGY is required in the Soul-life. The actual change of view-point needs no exertion at all, but merely enlightenment.

Whilst it is of the utmost importance to seek the cause of disease, it is perhaps more imperative to set out to discover the goal or purpose the ailment is unconsciously serving. With such a discovery, those early training formulae become exposed to the patient, that are responsible for the nature of the goal and the method of its achievement.

Every patient comes to treatment with a system of training formulae or rigid rules of life acquired in his early days. This inner disposition forms the very foundation of his attitude towards life, of his attitude towards his fellow-beings, and above all, of the production of his symptoms. The object of treatment, therefore, is the releasing and breaking down of this disposition so antagonistic to life, or what amounts to the same thing, the substitution of a new "productivity" for the old rigidity. Thus do the training formulae govern the patient's attitude towards everyone, and therefore also towards the practitioner.

When the training formulae dictate that one must not confide in anybody, that one must make a good impression, and that one must secretly be superior to others, so will these characteristics inevitably work themselves out between doctor and patient, and indeed from the very first moment. The patient will try to make a good impression upon the doctor, but he will not unreservedly place his trust in him; he will even seek to make fun of him over some obscure point. If now the practitioner shows any signs of annoyance he is no true physician, but yet and in spite of the fact that psychotherapy has been established for a very long time now, many practitioners, even to-day, often sternly say to their patients: "If you do not place your entire confidence in me, we can get no further," or, "If you are going to behave in a dramatic manner just to impress me, I cannot do anything with you." Or even, "if you think you have the better of me, and if you are going to gain some fun at my expense, then we part company." Here the cure is doomed to failure right at the very start, as the practitioner does not understand that training formulae are governing his patient's attitude, as indeed, they are ruling his own.

An interesting point that is noted in practice is that those individuals who are powerfully extraverted are strongly inclined to suffer physical disturbances of function, whilst those who are exceptionally introverted suffer far more often from conditions of manias and phobias. It however, by no means follows that those who are behaving in an extraverted manner are behaving for *objective* purposes, in spite of their behaviour being of an objective nature. Objective behaviour can be just as much in the service of egocentric purposes as egocentric behaviour, but never VICE VERSA.

Let us remember then that health should not be the ultimate goal of existence, but the MEANS WHEREBY we can live more abundantly in the service of our fellow-men.

CHAPTER 25

THE LADY WITH A GOITRE

GOITRE IS not just a pain which none can see, but is an enlargement of the thyroid gland producing an unsightly swelling in the front of the neck which is visible to all and sundry, thus any improvement from treatment can be actually seen without one having to rely solely on the statement of the patient. This makes the case, which I am now about to relate, all the more convincing.

The patient is a woman, somewhat illiterate but most intelligent. She knew little or nothing about the functions and powers of the unconscious mind, and I took care not to approach her case on these lines, at least at the outset. All she wanted was that something practical should be done to effect a reduction of the ugly growth, which was so disfiguring to an otherwise very attractive person. She was a down-to-earth kind of individual in some ways, yet hypersensitive in others, but open to learn.

Leaving aside the psychogenic aspect for the nonce, purely physical treatment consisting of osteopathy and nature cure methods were resorted to.

The improvement that was effected was indeed most gratifying, so much so that the patient felt that she was nearly cured and decided to cease coming for treatment, towards the end of which I began instructing her in matters of the mind and the tremendous influence it exercised upon the body and its functions. By this time I knew my lady, and I had therefore reason to know that the fundamental cause of her complaint had not been removed. Notwithstanding this I refrained from persuading her to continue treatment, which would have been bad policy seeing that she had definitely made up her mind to get along on her own.

It therefore occasioned me no surprise to see this patient back in my consulting room about four months later with a goitrous throat worse than ever.

Having previously given her some instruction about the mind and the influence it can have on the matter, I asked her point blank what kind of an emotional upset she had suffered recently? This was her rejoinder: "You know that awful, detestable sister-in-law of mine, of whom I told you when I was with you before, well, we had a hell of a quarrel a week or so ago." Then she used these figures of speech: "Everything that woman utters sticks in my *throat.*" And, "I cannot swallow what *she* says."

Here I must remark that the primitive is in all of us whether we be civilised or uncivilised. Racial memories from down the ages seem to be impressed in the very depths of our being, some affecting us may be, and some not. Now, at one time it was believed that the entry into the soul of a man was by way of the mouth and throat. Our patient evidently could not accept into her soul the terrible utterances of her sister-in-law, hence they stuck in her throat, and being stuck there she obviously could not swallow them and, added to this, she certainly had no wish to.

Is it any wonder, then, that under such extreme emotional stress, the throat should swell up? Let the reader try this simple experiment: act and feel and say with emotion "It sticks in my throat." He will almost at once be made aware of a sensation of restriction in the throat, as if there were indeed an obstruction in it. This sensation will remain for a few minutes and even longer depending upon the degree of emotion put into words. The feeling in the throat is that experienced by some after swallowing a pill with difficulty. Now think of what a real, intense emotion that puts up a strong obstruction to wicked utterances entering the soul, can do to the throat and to the whole organism for that matter.

My patient, being a most intelligent being, as previously stated, was not slow to grasp the significance of my remarks for she at once recognised the purpose of the primitive defence mechanism her unconscious mind had adopted to stop the evil at the very entrance to her soul. But such emotional reactions sustained over a period of time left their mark in the swelling of the throat. Tenseness in any part of the body will interfere with proper circulation of the blood to the detriment of the tissues involved.

It is immaterial whether the theories expounded herein are considered by some to be "baloney" or not, the fact remains that the throat enlargement of my patient disappeared, and very quickly at that, after enlightenment came to her through my explanations. Because she offered no more resistance to her sister-in-law's bitter words, they just passed "over" her, and as she bore no resentment as previously, she was no longer all tensed up. Not long after the attitude of the sister-in-law towards my patient changed for the better.

Those who cannot believe what is meant by saying that "mind influences matter" should think again. My own experiences compel me to prefer to say, with Faraday, that "nothing is too wonderful to be true."

CHAPTER 26

THE MAN WITH AN OBSESSION FOR PLAYING WITH WATER

IN MY record files is an old case card which has written on it under the caption of complaint "Patient has an obsession for playing with water." This case provides me with material for an article that may not only prove interesting and instructive to many readers, but may also serve to "ring a bell" in those who suffer from other compulsory acts, or a tendency thereto, and thus this article could be of immense value in helping to effect a release.

It is really surprising how many there are among us who are more or less afflicted with all kinds of compulsions such as having to count things, or when sitting in a car being under a "must" to add up the figures on the number plates of cars in front. Then there are some who must avoid stepping on the cracks in the pavement, not to mention those individuals, perhaps running into many hundreds, who are "forced" by some inner power to bypass a ladder rather than go under it. And so on, and so on ...

I find that by relating suitable cases to patients, who are under psychological examination, many respond in a most remarkable manner, in that something in the case history I am relating strikes straight home: and here and there an instantaneous cure is brought about. It can be looked upon as a short cut method, which reduces the number of treatments, but it certainly is not always effective, although it generally enables the patient to talk more freely and gives him greater hope of being freed from his mental trouble.

Now to the case which prompted me to write this article.

The patient was a working man in his forties referred to me by a vicar of the Church of England, who said that he would be responsible for the fees.

After I had recorded the particulars of this man's medical history I asked him to give details of his present complaint, and this is what he related:

"When I get home in the evenings after my day's work, I feel compelled to go to the kitchen sink, turn on the tap and there I just have to play with water for some time. I cannot leave it alone, then leaving the sink I go about the house wiping everything with my bare, wet hands. I go over my person in the same way stroking my shoes, furniture and things with rapid movements of my hands. This goes on for 'hours' at a time."

After listening to this description of his compulsive acts, I uttered this remark: "What you are doing is *to you* a 'reasonable'

115

thing. Your intelligent and conscious self does not think so, and you are right from the point of view of what is considered to be normal behaviour. You believe that this compulsive act of yours is a 'daft' thing to do, and so do all the others who witness your unusual conduct; but let me say this: nothing ever happens without a cause, a reason, and when we discover this, as I hope to, you will readily see that what you have been and are doing in this strange way is 'reasonable' in so far as it is consistent with the cause behind the urge, but when you become conscious of the cause then the urge to play with the water and to wipe will disappear, for you will recognise that these acts are now *un*reasonable, for they can no longer serve the unconscious purpose of the original cause which had been relegated to the depths of the unconscious mind, and was operative from there."

This clarification greatly comforted and encouraged the patient, and it at once established a most favourable transference or rapport, which latter term I much prefer.

Analysis was now proceeded with, but only the essential details of it can be given here, which will suffice the purpose of this article.

On the patient being asked to describe some of his earlier experiences in life he immediately started on those he had had as a stretcher bearer in the Royal Army Medical Corps in world war 1914-18. When carrying out his duties as a stretcher bearer in France he had to cross a wide stretch of water to fetch in the wounded. This water was not deep, but on his return journey through it to the first aid post he felt, for some unaccountable reason, safe from the "Jerries'" shells, and this feeling of security was enhanced because, in some inexplicable way, it was shared by his comrades.

This confession brought up into my mind the following thoughts: "Water to this man signifies safety. It appears to him as a protective agent. From what, I asked myself does he to-day wish to be protected, so that he is now compelled to occupy himself so intensely for long periods at a time with water and in such a ridiculous manner?" These thoughts led to my putting the query to the patient: "What is water for?" He naturally replied: "To drink and to wash with, to cleanse." I then requested him to go through the characteristic movements he made over the furniture and his person. "What are you doing?" I asked. "I am wiping away something." "What?" I responded. "I really don't know" he answered.

At a subsequent sitting I questioned him as to what disease he was afraid of. "None to my knowledge," he replied, but he disclosed soon after, that when a lad he had had the bad habit of rubbing his cheek. This caused his mother on many occasions to remonstrate with him about it and the patient now remembered

116

that his mother had a mortal dread of cancer, and she was constantly telling him in an emotionally charged voice that if he kept on rubbing his cheek in the way he did, he would certainly get cancer of the face.

Such admonitions do not always appear to make a deep conscious impression during the tender years of childhood, but the suggestions conveyed can reach the unconscious mind, and be firmly registered and rooted there, so that it only requires an appropriate stimulus or shock in later life to bring into actual existence the emotion appertaining to (but not the memory of) its origin, which emotion can then find expression in peculiar behaviour such as the playing with water under an inner compulsion.

The patient now clearly realised that as water in France had "proved" to be a protective agent making him feel safe from the enemy's fire, so somehow water became connected in his mind with protecting him from the dreaded cancer, and as water is cleansing he was wiping away cancer from things around him and from his own person. This realisation caused such a strong emotional discharge that he declared he felt freed from his former obsession. Memory by itself unaccompanied by the emotion attached to it is ineffective in bringing about a cure.

A week later our patient called to report and gave this glad news: "Only once after the last treatment, on the next day, did I experience the urge to go to the kitchen sink, but when I had turned on the water, I asked myself what do I want to do here? There was simply nothing in me to respond. There was no reaction, except one of great joy at my release." He was completely cured of his obsession, i.e., when he realised that in using water for wiping he was fulfilling an unconscious motive to wash away cancer. This then, *in the circumstances* obtaining at the time, was to him, a perfectly "reasonable" thing to do although he was obviously not motivated by conscious reasoning.

Now, when he was made fully aware of what was at the back of it all, viz: a great fear of contracting cancer, and on it being pointed out to him that this disease, so far as it is known, is not contageous, not infectious, not even hereditary he saw the "unreason" of his former obsessional acts with the water and wiping.

Did not Pontius Pilate call for a basin of water wherewith to wash away something disagreeable? But whereas Pilate knew why he was doing it, and knew of the symbolism that was behind the act of his washing his hands, our patient was quite unaware of his. To the conscious mind they were purposeless actions, which however, had a definite unconscious purpose behind them. But both men had been using the same medium of water, the one to wash away his sense of guilt, and the other to wash away the disease of cancer so keenly *felt* to be lurking on everything.

Apart from the practical uses of that wonderful element, water, so common, so ubiquitous, it plays a great part in spiritual matters. Just ponder on the baptismal water of the river Jordan, the holy water in the church font, the blessed holy water of the Roman Catholic Church, the spiritual curative power of the water at Lourdes shrine. Look up the second book of Kings, chapter five, wherein Naaman is told by Elisha to go and wash in Jordan seven times so that he may be cleansed of his leprosy. The Bible is full of references to the Divine-healing power of water; and even the rain falls from "heaven."

CHAPTER 27

THE BOY WITH THE INTRACTIBLE COUGH

A BOY of fifteen years of age had suffered from a very severe, hard cough for about eighteen months, which would not yield to any form of medical treatment. The family doctor, and the specialists consulted, were frankly puzzled by the condition and by the lack of response to the therapies prescribed.

The lad's father now decided to bring his son to an osteopath, but examination did not reveal anything osteopathically diagnostic. I was thus moved to seek the cause in the boy's psyche, as I felt convinced that this chronic cough was psychogenic in origin.

Before me was a bright, intelligent youngster with an excellent family background. The first question I put to him was did he like school. "Oh yes" he replied "I like school very much indeed, but for ... " "But for what?" I interrupted and he replied: "Latin and mathematics. I loathe and detest these two subjects." I then asked: "Have you noticed whether there were occasions when you coughed more than on others?" Pausing a few minutes before replying, as if in deep thought, he exclaimed with growing astonishment "Now I come to think of it my cough is worse on Tuesdays and Fridays." "Why on these particular days?" I queried. "I have no idea." he said.

After a brief pause I followed up my previous question with this query: "On what days do you have instruction in Latin?" "On Tuesdays" he responded. The boy was now intensely alert. I continued: "and of course on Fridays you have tuition in mathematics." "Yes" he said. By this time he was fully alive as to what I was getting at, for he asked with great feeling: "Do you think that I have been deliberately 'putting on' this cough? Do you think I could produce a cough like this at will." "Of course not," I countered. Neither could he, of that I was certain.

Now I asked the lad to go back in his mind to eighteen months ago, before the severe cough had become established. He related that he had caught a heavy cold and was confined to bed with a high temperature; and then said: "Come to think of it, it was at the time of the examinations in the dreaded subjects of Latin and mathematics. I recovered from the cold but not from the cough, which has persisted right up to the present, more especially on the mornings of Tuesdays and Fridays." I then asked him, what occurred on these mornings when he coughed so badly. "Oh," he replied, "my mother would say that I could not go to school that day, and on a recent occasion my cough was so severe that both my parents said that there was nothing for it but that I should remain at home." Soon after he had told me this he had to admit that the relief he felt was so great that for the rest of the day *he did not cough once.*

Just two treatments on these lines sufficed to clear up the cough completely, which did not return—much to the amazement of himself and of his parents.

Now that the boy was fully conscious of the *purpose* his cough was serving it was not in his nature to play the malingerer and use his cough as an excuse to stay at home in order to escape attending his Latin and mathematics classes respectively. His unconscious motive was revealed to him and this, in his case, effected the cure and enabled him to take his Latin and mathematics in his stride, which in turn raised his morale very considerably. Thus was a truly beneficent cycle established.

CHAPTER 28

A COLD IS NOT AN ILLNESS

As I do not wish to be thought guilty of plagiarism I must say that this article is based upon one that I read in a German periodical some time ago, and credit must, therefore, be given to Dr. Heinz Graupner, the orginator and author of the ideas upon which I have elaborated.

The doctor started his article with a plea that his readers, in as far as they may be suffering from a cough or a running head-cold, will not be nettled with him because of the title of his article. When he stated that a cold is not an illness he did not for one minute mean to imply that those afflicted with a cough or cold in the head are perfectly well, when they simply cannot exist without a handkerchief or are unable to speak a complete sentence without coughing; nor did he wish to imply that they imagine their condition. Of course, they have caught a cold; but a cold is not an illness, but a release. This, however, will be a matter of indifference to the host of sufferers from colds whose numbers always increase in the winter months of each year. To them, a cold is a matter of *fact* and not of mere words. But, as Dr. Graupner puts it: "Is it not just the same as if a hunter were to say that he shot with the bolt of his gun and not with the cartridge?" As the bolt releases the bullet or shot in its flight, so does the cold release the running nose and cough.

This assertion that a cold is not an illness is, without doubt, of practical significance, for just as the cartridge lies harmless in the magazine of the gun so long as the trigger is not pressed, so colds do not become active when the body is protected.

Now, that is easier said than done. One is more prone to colds when windows and doors of our dwellings do not shut properly in the winter time, and when, through lack of coal, our heating is not so efficient as we might wish. In this respect, there are two groups of people who can teach us a thing or two.

One group catches cold very quickly because, say, a window pane is broken. The other group, however, has fewer head colds or bronchitis when living under spartan conditions than in those times when the central heating radiates a luxurious warmth. It is the same with many who move from the town to the country, substitute a stove for their central heating, and sleep in an unheated room. It is noticed that they usually have fewer colds after such a change. Who has not known of someone who, returning from the country to the town in winter and living in centrally-heated surroundings, has promptly caught a cold—and a very severe one at that?

Now, comfortable warmth and protection against colds do not in any way go hand in hand. Indeed, did not doctors discover this during the first world-trench-war? Out of one thousand men in the field who were subjected to bitter cold and wet there were only about four cases of inflammation of the lungs and eighteen cases of tonsilitis; while among the occupation troops living protected in houses there were about six cases of inflammation of the lungs and *thirty* cases of tonsillitis. Hence, it follows that one does not catch cold because the weather is cold or wet or because there is a draught.

Two things can help us to avoid catching cold so that illness need not develop:

First, there is always the much-praised hardening process. This requires our co-operation, and we shall not achieve this merely by the application of the (in most instances) much hated cold water, but by exposure to the *air*. He who, on arising in the mornings, exposes his nude body to the air with the windows wide open, even if it be only for a few minutes, will have gone a long way towards making himself immune to colds. Any feeling of coldness can be obviated by bodily movements; he may start to tidy up his bedroom, for example, which is better and more profitable than doing a set of boring exercises. But this exposure to the air must be carried out daily, even when the weather is not at all friendly.

Secondly, there is the avoidance of *anxiety* about catching cold. He who always thinks he is going to contract a cold or a cough has already half opened the door to the appropriate stimulus. The peasant goes out of a very warm kitchen across his yard to the stable in bitter weather without troubling to put on a coat or even thinking about it—it is just a matter of habit with him. But he does not take cold, in spite of the great change in temperature.

Yes, we can even go further and say catching cold is also a matter of *mood*. Whoever is depressed or in a bad humour catches cold much more easily.

This reminds the writer of something that Dr. Braithwaite, Psychiarist to the Ministry of Health, wrote in the *British Medical Journal*, of 2nd October, 1943, on the common cold:

"The following facts may be of interest to either sufferers from, or investigators of, the common cold:

"During the course of twenty-five years practice of psycho-analysis for the treatment of psycho-neurotics, I have observed in them:

1. A cold invariably occured in a particular emotional state.

2. The occurrence of a cold could be prognosticated whenever this state developed.

3. The cold could be aborted if a different emotional state could be produced in the course of treatment, or could be shortened if it had started.

4. Cold, wet, hunger, exhaustion, and a source of infection do not result in the development of a cold in the absence of the appropriate emotional state.

5. Cold 'proneness' disappears completely as a result of successful (psychological) treatment and does not return."

Dr. Braithwaite continues: "My experience demonstrates to me, at least, that the solution of the problem of the common cold lies in the sphere of preventive psychological medicine. The specific factor is psychological; the microbic one secondary."

Dr. Braithwaite's remarks on the common cold should certainly make one think, and they find full support in the introduction to the third edition of Dr. Flanders Dunbar's large book on *Emotions and Bodily Changes*, under the caption, "Cold Habit," from which the following is quoted:

"It is not customary to apply the psychosomatic approach to the problem of infectious diseases. Nevertheless, as Osler said: what happens to a patient with tuberculosis depends more on what he has in his head than what he has in his chest.

"It is well known that in epidemics there is always a percentage of those exposed who do not succumb to the disease. It is said that some persons have a higher resistance to infection than others, and this higher resistance cannot always be explained in terms of immunization. Resistance to disease is greatly modified by such factors as fatigue and the general physiological equilibrium of the body. As Cannon and many others have demonstrated, maintenance of the physiological equilibrium is a psychosomatic problem. Whether the psychic or the somatic aspect be considered primary, the real problem is to treat, first the patient, then the disease process, and only third, the symptom.

"Experiment shows that emotional stress seriously limits the ability of the organism to regain a stable equilibrium after it has been subjected to stress or injury. There could be no better illustration of this fact than the enormous difference in susceptibility to colds, and in rapidity of recovery, among different individuals. No adequate scientific description of the causation of colds can yet be given. A multitude of bacteria and viruses have been found in nose and throat cultures of patients with and without colds. Colds are of different types with different consequences. It is known that quite aside from psysiological susceptibility, there is such a thing as a cold habit or accident-proneness which somewhat parallels the accident habit or cold-proneness. Gladstone is reported to have suffered from 'diplomatic' colds which occurred regularly when he was required to speak in an unpleasant situation.

"Since no one can entirely escape exposure to the various agents which may cause colds, and since there is no known way of producing complete immunity against colds, the factors in human beings which may increase or decrease susceptibility to colds assume primary importance.

"Saul reported that fifteen patients unusually susceptible to colds or sore throat who were treated psychoanalytically for other reasons, following treatment became either entirely free from colds or acquired them extremely rarely. In these cases no other treatment such as vaccine, was given. This is a common experience. Sometimes brief psychotherapy directed towards the 'cold habit' seems to produce relative immunity from colds. But a marked improvement is almost always observed in patients susceptible to colds who have been subjected to a thorough psychoanalysis."

Look to your emotional state, then, immediately you become aware of having contracted a cold; but that certainly does not mean that the health precepts are to be ignored.

When Christ healed he said: "Go and sin no more."

CHAPTER 29

COLOUR THERAPY

OVER A long period of time scientists, philosophers, poets and artists have all concerned themselves with colours. Colour lore is as old as mankind itself, and, since it was discovered that white light, i.e., daylight, is composed of all the colours of the rainbow and which can be split up into each individual colour by means of a prism, physical researches of an exact nature have established the basis on which results of colour therapy can be obtained to-day.

A long way back in time colour lore differentiated "warm" and "cold" colours that exercise various external and internal influences upon our respective dispositions, and in this respect I now relate in support of the effects of colour rays upon all living organisms, a remarkable experience I had with a Mr. J. Deighton-Patmore, the grandson of the famous poet Coventry Patmore.

Many years have passed since I called upon this "Magician of Light," as he was then known, at his flat in Mayfair. He showed me his "vessels of light" as he called them. Switching off all the lights in the room with the exception of one, which to me, had the appearance of what I termed a tall "blanc-mange" or "ice-berg," having a sickly bluish white hue something like "dirty" moonlight, if I may so describe it. Mr. Deighton-Patmore had named it "The Ice Age Lamp." And how aptly named it was, for almost at once I experienced a disagreeable sensation of cold almost to the point of shivering, although the actual *temperature* of the room had not changed. It would seem that these "starchy bluish" rays had some alterative effect upon the heat-regulating centre in the brain, and this theory would appear to find confirmation in the following experience:

The "Ice Age" lamp was switched off and now the lamp known as the "Sun Bowl" switched on. I soon felt all aglow from the warm orange rays emitted. A little later I was asked to stand sideways with one cheek close to, but not touching the lamp. There was a definite sensation of warmth. I was then requested to press my cheek against the illuminated bowl; but I remember hesitating to do so believing that the bowl would be uncomfortably warm. However, to my great surprise it was quite *cool*. I was then asked to look into a mirror and to compare the colour of my two cheeks, to find that the cheek that was exposed to the direct rays of the orange lamp was of a deeper red than the other.

Whilst this "Sun Bowl" lamp was still illuminated I was requested to go down a passage, quite a distance from the lamp, and read a book of fairly small print. Here again was a surprise in that I could see how very clearly the print stood out in that peculiar subdued orange light, making the reading so easy, thus evidencing the great penetrating power. It is just because all this made such an impression upon me at the time so many years ago that I can recall the details with such facility.

Goethe, of course, was *the* great authority on colour, with whom the erstwhile dissenting experts had perforce to agree. In more modern times there was a Dr. E. D. Babbit, who wrote that encyclopaedic work, "The Principles of Light and Colour," and since then further research has been carried out by E. J. Stevens, M.Sc., M.A., and also by Dr. Starr-White.

Light travels at the inconceivable speed of 186,000 miles per second, and colour is light in its various rates of vibration; for example, it is said that red, at one end of the spectrum, has a wavelength of .0000256 of an inch, and violet at the other end, has a wavelength of .0000174 of an inch. Below red is the infra-red and the invisible heat rays; above blue is the ultra-violet and chemical rays.

When there are coarse vibrations we have sound. Below 32 down to about 16 impulses per second the ear detects each separate impulse. Above 32 a musical note is produced. The highest note the ear can register is in the region of 25,000 vibrations per second. When the vibrations become higher or finer then colour is manifested. These vibrations are now etheric and are no longer sound waves. The rate of vibrations of red is 450 trillions per second, and as the rate of vibrations increases so are the different colours seen. Each colour has a distinct unchangeable period of vibration. In contrast to the red, violet's rate of vibrations is 780 trillions per second. Beyond this rate then colour is no longer visible to the human eye. Now we have the ultra-violet and X-rays, etc. The former should be cautiously used; the latter not at all therapeutically, and the same goes for radium too, only more so.

The conclusions of E. J. Stevens are summed up in these words: "Colour-energy is as necessary as our meals in stimulating and maintaining our body activities. In fact, it is the colour-energy within the food elements, particularly within the minerals, that restores our health and happiness. We may obtain this vital colour-energy from all edible plant life." He became thoroughly convinced that colour possesses not only properties for maintaining the health of the body, mind and spirit, but also curative powers in disease conditions.

An Indian doctor by the name of Dinshah P. Chiandali, who works at the Spectrochromo-Institute in New Jersey, has written much which is of interst in his reports. This doctor does not speak of *diseases* as such, but only of "discord" or "disharmony" of the make-up of the human organism; hence a return to the harmonious working of the body-mind results in a cure. Those who seek to be cured by Dr. Chiandali are treated by him gratuitously, but only on the understanding that those patients who are cured by his methods become his pupils, and what is more, that they try to maintain their new-found health by using the powers that are inherent in colour.

Dr. Chiandali is of the opinion, and in this he is in agreement with other physicians who employ light and colour in their treatments, that a more far-reaching stimulating action lies in coloured light than is the case with white light—sunlight or artificial white light. He based his colour therapeutics upon the results of modern medicine and chemistry. "Disharmonious causes" are removed by stimulating the natural healing power of the organism by means of various colour rays. It goes without saying that such a healing method requires a thorough knowledge of chromotherapy.

Over many years of careful research and of laborious detailed work Dr. Chiandali arranged the prismatic colours into 12 grades, which he then subdivided into two groups, viz.:—One with a "content of yellow" and the other with a "content of blue." "Red" he named the "warm pole," "blue" the "cold pole." All illnesses that have a red colour, e.g., fevers, inflammations, blood poisoning, swellings, etc., indicate that as "red" is the WARM pole an excess of heat is present. Now, in order to restore the balance, the cold colour "blue" is necessary.

Chiandali also describes, inter alia, how wonderfully the colour possessing the opposite pole acts. Here is an illuminating example: A nine-year-old girl had sustained a "fatal" burn of the third degree. The child was admitted to the Women's Hospital, Philadelphia, where there is a colour therapeutic department. The resident physician at this hospital herself really believed that the case was absolutely hopeless, but in spite of this conviction she at once began to administer colour rays. The scarcely hoped-for wonder happened. Already, after the first day, the child had practically no more pain, and in the course of time, the wounds healed without leaving even a scar behind. Eight photographic exposures were made in order to show the curative process and to provide evidence of the cure.

There are two hundred and thirteen kinds of inflammation that are differentiated by doctors. Chandali cites them all, but adds that it is not essential to know them all, the main thing is that one should know to which "group" the disharmony belongs. Thus, for example, he restored the sight to a seventy-six year old blind woman because he was able to determine the cause of blindness and the correct therapeutic colour or colours required for the particular condition. It was a question of reducing the excitability of the nerves of the eye.

There are physicians also in Germany who employ colour-therapy with success. One of the most meritorious pioneers of light and colour was the head of the Scientific Association in Munich, a Professor Dr. Edwald Paul.

Those who are interested to the point of experimentation can watch the growth of the same species of plant under different coloured glass frames; and people whose work compels them to sit long hours at a desk or table could experiment with separate pieces of silk of different colours within easy reach of the vision. By occasionally glancing at them they will find a pleasant relief from eye strain.

Those who study at night should do so by an amber, orange or deep yellow light, as either of these colours is a mental stimulant. Then prior to going to bed for the night the student should look easily at a large piece of silk of natural green and finally blue, which colours are calming and counteract the stimulating effect of the amber, orange, or yellow.

CHAPTER 30

HEALING MAGNETISM

WHENCE originated the name "MAGNET?" The ancient Roman Plinius, who was famous as a naturalist, asserted that the name came from a shepherd who was called Magnes. One day he accidentally contacted a stone with his iron ferruled staff, when he found that the iron ferrule was sticking to it. Thus the lodestone or magnetic stone was discovered. From the magnetic stone originated the term mineral magnetism. The healing power magnetism, was so named because it had many similarities with the properties of mineral magnetism, namely in regard to the power of its lines of force.

The use of healing magnetism is certainly as old as mankind itself, and instinctively employed in very ancient times. Later healing magnetism was practised almost exclusively by the privileged priesthood, and was guarded as a strict secret. Especially in Egypt were the temples, with their halls for the sick, widely famous as curative establishments. Also the oracles in Greece were the revelations of magnetised, clairvoyant persons.

So mankind in general remained in ignorance of healing magnetism and its wonders for many thousands of years. The few initiates jealously guarded their treasured knowledge.

Only at the commencement of the 17th century did a shimmer of light of the awakening dawn appear after a long night.

Paracelsus, whose writing appeared in 1603 in Strasburg, gave the first significant pointer, and his successor van Helmont, dared to answer in regard to attacks on his magnetic cures in this way: "Whoever looks upon magnetic cures as the works of the devil must, by the same token, regard the causes of all magnetic phenomena as devil's magic." Sound logic, isn't it?

Magnetism, which is everywhere present, is nothing new apart from its name, but when it is used as a healing method—and a very valuable one at that—then certain over pious individuals with closed minds decry it and attribute the phenomenon to the power of the devil when it is used for curative purposes. Hypnotism and hypnotherapy come in for similar abuse by the unenlightened.

In these days of hurried living, eulogies are voiced abroad from time to time, about the latest methods of healing, which are near to being "infallible," and which promise mankind a superabundance of health, but alas only to be discarded because they do not come up to the tenth part of what has been claimed for them.

129

There can be no shadow of doubt that through the medium of herbs, biochemic and homœopathic remedies, striking cures can be achieved, as many who have thereby been restored to health can vouch for.

In order, however, that these methods of healing can be properly employed, it is essential that a precise diagnosis be arrived at, and should this prove to be erroneous, then all efforts on behalf of the patient in this direction become more or less futile, according also to the suggestibility of the patient. It is, naturally, the correct selection of the curative agent that is of fundamental importance which must not only be suitable for the type of particular ailment, but also appropriate to the type of the patient himself. If care be not taken here, the method employed may not be any use whatever, but indeed may even be injurious to the patient, and thus the last state may be worse than the first.

With the use of healing magnetism, however, no mistakes of this kind can arise.

The question may well be asked: "What then is this animal or human magnetism?" It may be considered as a kind of emanation to which has been given many different names, but the one that appeals to me most is odic or odylic force. It flows from every living soul in all directions being fine vibratory in nature. It is in the animals, plants and minerals and this subtle element is universal. It is especially sensed by those of a sensitive nature and who are in harmony with their surroundings.

It has been postulated that this force may be the result of the splitting of atoms into electrons and ions, and perhaps a disintegration into the finest ether. This living stream of power is composed of luminiferous substance, which as a matter of fact, has been demonstrated by Baron von Reichenbach and others working in this field. If, for the time being, we do not know the actual source of this power, we can at least recognise quite clearly the EFFECTS it produces in magnetic healing, which can be of a very striking nature indeed, as is evidenced by some who were seriously ill becoming well in a few hours after such treatment. A harmonious recovery can take place even in cases of long standing disease.

This transference of the peculiar odic force that is embraced in magnetism from one human being to another and the absorption of these restorative radiations by the patient, is without doubt, the surest and incontestable healing method extant, provided the patient and healer are in CONCORD—en rapport—with each other.

Suitable relaxation technique and suggestion may be employed to advantage for the establishing of this harmony where it is felt that this is weak or absent.

Healing magnetism is, fortunately, a very safe form of treatment, even when conducted by lay people, in that a diagnosis of the complaint is not essential, for it cannot and does not affect the good results that follow the treatment. This does not mean, however, that professional advice should not be sought in serious cases, but whatever the clinical diagnosis findings may be, there are no contraindications to magnetic treatment. No injurious effects or risks are to be feared from the use of this method whatever the medical history and present complaint of the patient may be.

It should be apparent that when the whole body is treated with human health-and-strength-giving radiations all the parts of the sick organism receive something of these rays, producing the harmony that is so necessary for the well-being of the individual under treatment. Hence, the result is not a mere improvement, but a complete cure in many cases, provided that destructive processes have not proceeded beyond repair so that they have become irreversable—and who can say for certain that they are!

Human radiations—the odic force— can actually be seen with the naked eye, not in the light of day, as they are not sufficiently luminous, but in a subdued light with a dark background.

If say the finger tips of each hand are spread out and are held opposite to each other about one inch apart emanations will be seen. They can be described as bluish or bluish-grey in colour and appear as strands of cobweb, or strands of chewing gum with a gossamer appearance in the spaces between the fingers. On the hands being separated the "lines of force" become thinner, and, naturally, as they are brought closer to each other, the strands appear thicker. A faint bluish mist can be discerned between the finger spaces, as already mentioned. If the fingers of each hand are moved up and down in conjunction with their opposites the strands will be seen to accompany the motions. They become more visible as the eyes become accustomed to the semi-darkness in which the finger movements are observed. It is just these radiations that emanate from the hands of the operator that act as a curative influence and become absorbed by the patient receiving the magnetic passes over his body generally, and over the part affected, in particular.

The healing touch has been known right down history, and most of us can sense the influence of the touch by different people in the common hand-shake. Such a lot can be conveyed to mind and body by touch, and when concentrated upon and used for healing purposes, it can and does have profound curative effects.

As a garment worn close to the skin can accumulate electricity and its discharge perceived by the crackling sound and seen by the naked eye in the form of sparks on removing the article of clothing, so I feel that the garment of Christ was saturated with healing magnetism when it touched the woman with the issue of blood on her putting her stretched out hand upon it, with a mind and body completely receptive to this wonderful power.

The *application* of this power is dealt with in the next chapter.

CHAPTER 31

THE PRACTICAL APPLICATION OF
HEALING MAGNETISM

READERS of my previous chapter on "HEALING MAGNETISM" will, naturally, wish to know how to apply the treatment to members of their families, as well as to their friends and others, who could be helped by this method.

The following instructions will enable them to try their hand at what has proved to be a most pleasant and effective therapy, when correctly done in faith and with a genuine desire to aid sufferers to be relieved and cured of their physical and mental troubles.

First have the patient placed in the "magnetic" position, which is, when he is sitting, having his back to the north, so that he will be facing the south. It is preferable, however, to have him lie down on a bed or sofa, the head of which should be towards the north and the foot to the south whenever this can be arranged. Incidentally this position of the bed is not only recommended for the sick, but also for the healthy and for those who otherwise find it difficult to get off to sleep at nights.

With the patient in the sitting position the operator takes hold of both of his hands with the thumbs against thumbs for about one minute. Then he commences with the long magnetic strokings. Begin these strokings or passes very slowly with both hands; first over the centre of the forehead moving the hands outwards, passing them over the eyebrows, temples and down each side of the neck continuing down on the right and left sides of the body respectively to over the toes and beyond otherwise the effect of the downward stroking will be lost. Repeat the movements as before a number of times. The treatment can be given either by contacting the patient's body with a light touch during the downward strokings with outspread fingers slightly bent, so that they are pointing more or less downwards, or the hands may be held about an inch or so away from the body. Each full length stroking should take about thirty seconds. Usually from seven to fourteen passes are made. After a short pause the strokings are to be repeated until an abatement of the trouble takes place. The effect of the treatment is enhanced when the patient is only lightly clad.

The magnetic strokes are sensed mostly as a soft draught, as if a cool current of air was coming through a straw. Immediately after the completion of the treatment the patient should be allowed to rest in a quiet room. It has been found that a practitioner who is endowed with strong magnetic powers can work successfully upon patients at a distance.

When treating it is advisable not to fix the eyes upon those of the subject with a staring gaze, as this could cause him some embarrassment.

The operator must always remember to treat the left side (negative) of the body with his right hand (positive), and the right side (positive) with the left hand (negative), because according to the law in nature, similar poles are not compatible, whereas dissimilar poles are. The above directions apply to the treatment of the patient in the supine position, but when he is lying face downwards, i.e., prone, he is to be treated by the operator with his hands crossed in order to ensure the correct polarity, so that the downward strokings are made with crossed hands. This applies to self-magnetisation in so far as it can be done. Anyone can free himself from pain from his own body in the front, by treating it with arms crossed. Note, the mind must constantly be centred upon the parts under treatment.

Baron von Reichenbach lays great stress upon avoiding using the same poles, i.e. negative-negative, positive-positive, although it is possible, in some cases, to relieve pain by not observing this rule, but it is better to stick to it by employing opposite poles.

Magnetic results are not only achieved by strokings or passes along the body or over the head, but also by the laying on of hands, by gentle blowing on the affected part or parts, and also by the use of magnetised substances.

The laying on of hands is a very ancient practice, and is, in many cases, highly curative. Every mother instinctively knows this when she is moved to place her hands upon the feverish brow of the sick child; but let her heed this advice: place the right hand on the chest and the left hand upon the forehead. This will help to sooth the child and to reduce the fever. Should the mother not be successful in this, then let one other member of the family or friend try. He or she may be blessed with more magnetic healing power than the mother, who may be too emotionally upset herself, and therefore drained of energy. Adults suffering from headaches can best be relieved by the laying on of hands by allowing the bent fingers of the right hand to rest upon the heart region and, at the same time, those of the left hand upon the forehead so that the thumb touches the bridge of the nose.

The magnetic force flows the most from the thumb and middle finger, which has been confirmed by many highly sensitive individuals. They have clearly seen the magnetic radiations emanating from the finger tips, which they described as an extremely fine, bluish mist surrounding the fingers and ascending like a vapour.

133

Every child, and adult for that matter, blows on his hurt hand to alleviate the pain. Here again we see instinct at work. A gentle but concentrated breathing upon a painful spot often works quicker, in some cases, than even magnetic strokings. Blowing several times on one side of the forehead to the other has proved to be an effective remedy for a stubborn headache. If one blows gently and repeatedly over the inflamed parts of erysipelas the redness has been seen to subside. The heat disappears and, it is claimed, often a dangerous brain inflammation can be prevented by this simple procedure.

In addition to magnetic strokings and blowing on the body it is deserving of mention that any substance can be magnetised by this method, and then used for healing purposes. For example, a silk handkerchief can be magnetised by blowing strongly upon it, and also by stroking it in one direction from above downwards. It is then to be fixed to the affected part by means of a bandage. It will be active continuously.

Among all the substances of Nature water is the most suitable in every way for the purpose of magnetic healing. Magnetised water is considered to be a universal remedy, and acts just as efficiently internally by drinking it, as it does when employed externally in the form of compresses, ablutions and baths. Severe vomiting can be allayed by drinking half a glass of magnetised water. In burns, cuts, contusions, sprains, cold water compresses that have been magnetised by stroking without direct contact by the fingers, are to be employed. Results are usually quicker than when the cold water compress is applied without first being magnetised. So speaks the voice of experience!

A bottle or a glass of water is magnetised by holding the glass on the finger tips of the left hand for a couple of minutes and, at the same time, holding the finger tips of the right hand over the opening. A bath, with the head end towards the north, where this is possible, is magnetised by slowly stroking quite close to the surface of the water with both hands about seven times. Care must be exercised that the strokings are made in one direction only, the arms being carried back in a wide sweep well away from the water to the starting point at the head of the bath. This is to obviate neutralisation. Complaints in small localised areas should be treated by circular movements of the finger tips. In cases of abdominal troubles the spread-out fingers of both hands are to be held over the affected region until no pain on palpation can be elicited. This treatment is to be followed by stroking from the pit of the heart to the feet.

Much more could be written upon this fascinating subject, but I shall conclude by citing an extraordinary experiment that was made on a young girl by a continental magnetopath of medical repute, and its result:

One day the girl complained to her mother about a foot trouble. The sufferer received magnetic treatment from a magnetopath when she fell asleep, which is not unusual. On finishing the treatment it occurred to the magnetopath to make a magnetic barrier across the centre of the room. He did not mention this to the girl or to the mother, but proceeded to make passes with his finger tips across the room; then he sat down near a window with the "magnetic barrier" between him and the girl, who lay on the sofa, which was so positioned that she could not see him, but even if she had been awake the girl would not have known that a magnetic obstruction had been made. When she did awake she felt quite free of her foot complaint, she put on her hat and coat and prepared to leave. Then the magnetopath from his seat near the window called out: "Now, Miss Mary come and shake hands before you go." "Willingly" she replied, and started to go to him, as she came to the place where the magnetic barrier had been set up she fell backwards and stumbled to the floor with a cry. The magnetopath quickly raised the ban by a counterstroke.

"What happened?" asked the girl. It was explained to her that a magnetic "fence" had been created across the centre of the room. She was then asked to say what she had felt. She replied that it was as if she had suddenly come up against an invisible wall.

Now this phenomenon is none the more remarkable than that of the cloud-dispersal demonstration by Dr. Rolf Alexander which took place on 12th September, 1954, in Orillia, Ontario, Canada by the power of his *thought* only. Eleven successful demonstrations of this kind were given under test conditions on Hampstead Heath, London, one of which was filmed and many still photographs taken, proving the power of mind over matter, and in this regard I recommend the reader to obtain the two books written by Dr. Rolf Alexander viz: *"The Power of the Mind—the System of Creative Realism,"* and *"The Mind in Healing."* *

Magnetic treatment does not appear to be much practised in this country of ours; it is perhaps scarcely known, which is more the pity, but some time ago I did hear of a Mr. Brook who evidently possessed an unusual amount of magnetism in his make-up, which he usefully employed on the Queen's horses and on others. He called the method "impulse change." He lays the tips of his fingers on the animal's withers for the passing of impulses into the nervous system of the creature and indeed of humans too. This creates conditions conducive to better performance all round.

---

* *"The Power of the Mind."* Published by T. Werner Laurie Ltd., London.

"The Mind in Healing." Published by Odhams Press Ltd., Long Acre, London. 18s. each.

Animals are very susceptible to magnetic treatment, and that would explain, to some extent, Mr. Brook's undoubted success in the treatment of horses by his gift of imparting "Impulses" of a beneficial nature. Many people too must have been greatly helped by him as a practising psychotherapist in Harley Street.

Readers who would like to pursue this subject further could not do better than read Germain Berder's most unusual book *"Your Hands can help to Heal you,"* in addition to the two books by Dr. Rolf Alexander already referred to.

CHAPTER 32

DISSEMINATED SCLEROSIS
SOME HELPFUL SUGGESTIONS

IT IS the purpose of this chapter to describe certain drugless treatments, which have given some very encouraging and progressive results, in spite of the fact that disseminated sclerosis is considered to be incurable by the medical profession all over the world. Cases have been recorded which have been cured or at least permanently improved, the progress of the disease having been arrested either spontaneously or it could reasonably be attributed to the therapy employed.

It must be frankly admitted, however, that remissions of symptoms during the course of the disease, do take place, with or without treatment, so that the patient's hopes rise only to be dashed as recurrence of the old and sometimes new symptoms appear sooner or later.

If the patient is under treatment and an improvement sets in, one is tempted to give credit to the treatment, and in some cases, justifiably so, the improvement showing itself in say a steadier gait, perhaps more often than not in spite of the treatment and not necessarily because of it.

It is, therefore, difficult to assess the efficacy of at least orthodox therapy for the effect of drugs can be most deceiving.

This is what Dr. Glueck of Germany has to say about the treatment of disseminated sclerosis:
"Of all the allopathic methods that of injections should be specially avoided in the treatment of this disease, such being solely a matter of experiment causing more damage than benefit, and in any case, can never cure this complaint. Only a strict natural way of living can arrest the disease and bring about an improvement. The diet must be exclusively vegetarian, without eggs, ordinary cheese or salt."

But more about the diet question later.

The exact cause of D.S. is not yet known, but it is obvious that there is some disturbance of the circulatory system, and any method that can effect an improvement will, of course, be to the great benefit of the patient. Remember also that the blood, that life-giving stream, is made up from the food we eat.

Dr. Aschner, author of "Technik der Konstitutionstherapie" writes (I now translate): "It is always worth while in diseases of the spinal cord, such as multiple sclerosis, to employ cantharidin plaster. Agreeable surprises are experienced on occasions. On the advice of a foreign doctor a large cantharidin plaster was placed over the region of the lower thoracic vertebrae and continued for a lengthy period. The man, to the astonishment of all, became mobile once again and could follow his occupation."

It does not require a trained, scientific mind in medical matters to recognise the very great importance of a blood-stream that is in itself not only chemically balanced, but also unhampered in its flow through the body. It is an axiom that only with proper uninterrupted circulation can we have bodily and mental health. Unless fresh blood of sufficient quantity and QUALITY is brought to circulate within, and is drained from the afflicted areas of the body, these areas cannot become normal. On the other hand, it is a physiological law that no part of the body can become diseased if it has its waste material removed and receives the adequate quantity and quality of blood.

It is quite evident that micro-organisms are not the primary cause of disease, but are merely secondary invaders on a suitable soil. In normalising disease conditions, Nature can be assisted only in her own way, in which sustained circulation is the most important factor. Note that it is not the ONLY factor.

Most degenerations, and these include also the NERVES, may be attributed to faulty nutrition. We shall attend to nutrition presently. What we are concerned with at the moment is how to improve the circulation. One of the most effective means in accomplishing this is what is known as the Cupping Therapy, the technique of which is fully described in Chapter 4. By employing this method the circulation to and through the SPINAL CORD and adjacent ganglia is increased, controlled and improved, providing new blood and removing toxic blood from diseased areas. Hence its value in treating Disseminated Sclerosis.

If the blood stream is not nourished by the proper food, the blood is unable to nourish the cells of the body, including the cells of the spinal cord, resulting in malnutrition and poor health. Therefore, if the properly nourished blood does not reach, in sufficient quantity, all areas owing to a deficient circulation, how may we then expect to enjoy good health?

The cupping method relieves the congestion and proves stimulating and invigorating. Treating over any morbid area diverts the blood from the underlying tissues to the surface, diminishing the congestion of the inflamed nerves or organs, enabling them to approach normality. It is the most efficient mechanical means for enabling reparative processes to take place through an improved blood supply.

The great advantage of the cupping treatment is that it can be used as a home treatment by any adult member of the family whose near relative is afflicted with this dread disease of D.S.

Another promising treatment is known as the Super-heating

measure: but for this the patient would have to be prepared to go to Germany, to the Weserbergland-Clinic, Hoster/Weser. The head physician of the clinic is Professor Dr. Lampert, whose book "Ueberwaermung als Heil-Mittel" (Super-heating as a Curative Measure) is published by the Hippokrates-Verlag Marquardt and Cie, Stuttgart, which firm has kindly given me permission to quote from it. Dr. Lampert writes (I now translate): ". . . According to our present-day knowledge one sees in Multiple sclerosis of the brain and cord a pronounced focal disease of the central nervous system, which is not hereditary, although it can be found in isolated families. An extraordinary slight contagious infection by an, up to now, unknown micro-organism is *assumed* to be the cause of the disease. (Notice the word 'assumed'—Translator.)

"One working hypothesis for the treatment of this disease is as follows: We see in multiple sclerosis—as already mentioned—a chronic disease of infection which advances in stages. These stages are characterised by damage to and healing of the nerve network. In places where damage by toxins of the unknown excitor sets in (toxins in my view are due to faulty nutrition: Translator) there arises, as a healing reaction, a local, circumscribed inflammation, brought about by the specific defensive powers which, to be sure, do not always suffice to remove completely the damage caused. There takes place, therefore, either a local healing or a formation of a cicatrix in the network of nerves. Hence the old and proved principle should be observed in the treatment by physiotherapy, viz.: to bring about the acute state from the chronic condition, so that ultimate cure can take place. The aim must be to increase the specific defensive powers exactly as with paralyses, and when possible, to weaken the exciting agent or even kill it. To this end the super-heating method is most suitable. On the assumption that the exciting agent is sensitive to heat it is treated with high body temperatures. In this way 28 patients with disseminated sclerosis were superheated. Of these patients three remained free from their complaint from 8 to 10 years, so that they could follow their daily occupations; 19 were improved and capable of light work, whilst six remained un-influenced.

"It has been observed that often at the onset of the disease and long before severe symptoms have developed, patients react especially well to superheating. Weakness and severe fatigue in the legs as well as spastic paralysis have been seen to clear up. The weakness in the arms is checked with a dynamometer before and after treatment.

"Increased successes have been obtained by both the Americans and French by giving at least 20, and when possible, 30 super-heatings."

An initial course that can set off the development of D.S. can often be traced to a fall resulting in severe shocks to the system. Shock of any kind can be a strong factor in creating conditions that are conducive to nerve degeneration, hence psychotherapy particularly

139

in the form of hypnosis and hypnoanalysis is indicated. Dr. Flanders Dunbar, in his monumental work on "Emotions and Bodily Changes," writes: —

"In cases of multiple sclerosis, one is reminded of the command 'take up thy bed and walk' when one is able to make paralysed patients get up from their mattress graves. However, this requires much patience.

"A patient suffering from spastic spinal paralysis was unable to eat or hold himself erect. After a few periods of superficial hypnosis —which has to be repeated from time to time—he was able to comb his hair, change his shirt, eat, write, etc. It is unnecessary to point out what relief even improvements of this sort may be to such persons. . . .

"A patient with multiple sclerosis, bedridden for years, was subjected to superficial hypnosis. Even after the first session she was able to walk through a long corridor."

Professor Dr. L. Angel demonstrated on the 20th April, 1950, how a very considerable improvement was achieved in three cases of D.S. within a short time, in two of which a complete working capability was restored by hypnotherapy.

The longer I am in practice the more do I see that behind almost every disease there is an EMOTIONAL factor or factors operating. There is usually a history of severe shock, or a series of lesser shocks, or prolonged worry with emotional upsets and stresses. All these create mental tension resulting in body tension, and these tensions, in turn, cause all bodily functions and processes to become deranged with repercussions upon the mind. A disease arising out of these causes is termed psycho-somatic, psycho-genic and should be treated by psycho-therapy as well as by physical means.

Since we are here now on the theme of hypnotherapy, I feel sure that readers will profit greatly from perusing my book "The Healing 'Sleep'."*

There is not the slightest doubt that there exists in human make-up an inherent force or power, that when tapped, releases "SOMETHING" which brings about "miraculous" cures, and it seems just as certain that there is a "Something"—"The Unknown Self," as Dr. Groddeck puts it, that creates conditions that are conducive to disease.

Now we come to the all-important matter of nutrition.

A German country physician, Dr. Evers by name, had the idea to feed a paralysed young woman, for whom the medical profession could do no more, with GERMINATING wheat grain and rye. Guided by an instinctive feeling he prescribed a special raw diet, which he thought would be suitable to effect a change for the better in the

*Published by Health Science Press at 12s. 6d.

woman's metabolism, or in other words, to call forth new powers which would effectively reduce the destructive processes affecting her nervous system.

The patient, whose life was soon to end, recovered. Many believed this a coincidence, but further equally striking results were reported.

Dr. Evers explains that years of faulty food, together with other factors, causes the central nervous system to become unstable. The other factors can be an accident causing severe shock, a bad bout of influenza, prolonged digestive and mental disturbances.

As an excess of food which is faulty in its composition creates an accumulation of toxins, a total reform in one's dietetic habits is imperative. In the first rank stands the GERMINATING grains of wheat and rye, as well as raw foods, viz.: fruits and vegetables in the form of salads.

To germinate the wheat and rye first cleanse the grains of the last harvest, then mix together in equal parts. Place in a bowl and, late in the evening, pour cold water over the mixture so that it is well covered. Early in the following morning drain off the water and leave the grain without water during the day. Then in the late evening cover again with fresh water and so on. Continue this day after day until germination sets in. It should not be allowed to proceed until the shoots are too long, otherwise the mixture will not taste good. It is best for the grain to be in a temperature of 57 to 64 degrees Fahrenheit and be covered over with muslin or cheese cloth.

Germination makes the grain softer so that it is easier to chew. The germination should take place in 3 to 5 days. Every morning, midday and evening the grain should be shaken in a sieve and swilled thoroughly with water so that the resulting yeast and acid bacilli are removed, as otherwise the taste will be affected. The germinated grain can perhaps best be eaten with coarse oatmeal, good quality milk, Yoghourt, goat or cream cheeses. About 18 months ago I had the privilege of meeting a Dr. Selzer, who is a specialist in the treatment of Disseminated Sclerosis on Nature Cure Lines. He conducts a most attractive establishment situated in the beautiful Black Forest, the address being Kurhotel Berghof Schönmunzach in Murgtal, Schwarzwald, Germany.

Dr. Selzer was visiting one of the leading Nature Cure Homes in England, and I acted as his interpreter. He explained his methods, which included a special dietetic régime and showed a series of films of his patients in different stages of the disease and in various stages of recovery. The series of films was so arranged that one could easily see the progressive improvement of each patient, i.e., "before" and "after" treatment had commenced. This was indeed most striking and convincing and gave evidence that a more positive attitude should be taken towards this "incurable" disease, but all the time exercising a cautious optimism.

There is in practice in Budapest a Hungarian doctor whose name is Franz Andreas Völgyesi, who, in my opinion, is one of the greatest authorities on hypnosis and hypnotherapy. I have read his two erudite works, which have been translated from the Hungarian language into German. The respective titles are: "Hypnosetherapie and Psychosomatische probleme" and "Die Seele is Alles" (The Mind is everything).

He has stated that even in severe organic diseases striking results have been achieved by hypnotherapy, so that it has been possible to improve both physically and mentally those suffering from disseminated sclerosis and Parkinson's disease, and in many cases these patients could carry out their various occupations independently over many years.

The director of the psychiatric and neurological Clinic of the University of Budapest, Professor B. Horányi has also testified how remarkably easier the gait becomes in patients who are victims of Parkinson's disease and how much more co-ordinated are their movements after treatment by hypnosis, and by other psychotherapeutic measures.

Another professor, Dr. L. Angyal at the above-named clinic, demonstrated in April, 1950, what a very considerable improvement was achieved in a very short time in three cases of disseminated sclerosis by suggestion even in the waking state, and in two cases there was even a complete restoration of the ability to work again.

If we wish to gain health, or anything else in life for that matter, we must be willing to accept in full the means whereby it can be attained.

It is the earnest hope of the writer of this chapter that the information and advice contained in it will turn out to be the "means whereby" sufferers from this crippling, soul-destroying disease of disseminated sclerosis will find relief, a near-cure, or even a cure.

CHAPTER 33

HEALING EARTH

IT WILL readily be conceded that anything that will enhance the *general* health of the body and mind will also exercise a beneficial influence upon any "specific" or "local" disease.

For this reason I feel justified in writing this chapter on the value of Healing Clay.

All living things have developed out of the crust of our earth, including man himself, life being maintained by the earth's various constituents as well as by cosmic forces acting and reacting upon the earth. It should then not be surprising, or difficult to understand, how a certain kind of soil can possess healing properties when taken internally, or if applied externally as compresses and packs.

In these days of artificial fertilisers and poisonous sprays, our fruits and vegetable foods must, as a consequence, be deficient in minerals so essential to our well-being. These, fortunately, can, to some extent, be made good by taking internally certain kinds of "primitive" soil in the form of clay or earth of volcanic origin. The taking of "Healing Earth" can be looked upon as a biochemic radium cure, as will be made clear later.

RADIOACTIVITY OF SOILS:

Professor J. Stoklasa of Prague once referred to the extraordinary favourable effect the radioactivity of our soil had upon the life therein and, therefore, upon the soil upon which the plant-world grew. He stated that radium was present in all soils.

In order that he could measure the quantity of radium in a given soil he named a unit, which amounted to one-thousandth of a milligram in 1,000 kilos of soil (that would be according to homoeopathic standards an attenuation of 12 X, an attenuation which is often exceeded in homoeopathic and biochemic practice).

He ascertained that soils which have evolved out of rock of volcanic origin possess a far stronger radioactivity than those formed of chalk, sandstone and other sedimentary deposits. Soils that have arisen from granite contain, for example, 2.58 of the aforementioned unit, and those from recent volcanic rocks—trachyte, basalt, etc.—somewhat less. In soils of diluvial origin, to which belong the various clays used as a remedy, only 0.46 of the above unit of radium is present.

From this it will be seen that the soils of volcanic origin are more potent than those others. The healing earth of Swiss origin is a disintegration of volcanic rocks of porphyritic constituents.

143

According to Professor Stoklasa it contains 2.32 parts of radium of the stated unit; i.e., *five times* as much as diluvial clay.

Searching observations have shown that the dosage for a favourable action of the healing earth used internally depends upon its *homoeopathic* radium content.

When considering radioactivity it should be mentioned that radium radiates three kinds of rays which are differentiated by the Greek letter or sign, *alpha, beta, gamma* of which the first is of special interest in that it can harm the oxidation process in our blood, whilst the mild *beta and gamma* rays are of importance for the organism.

It is known that the terrestrial rays, i.e., the rays that emanate from our earth's crust, belong to the *gamma* group. Hence we have to thank, above all, the *gamma* rays of radium for the curative effect of the healing earth, besides its other components.

A lady had for many years sought help of several doctors for a complaint, to which all kinds of names had been given, and which had not been successfully diagnosed, but after taking healing earth masses of pin-worms were eliminated. These had been at the bottom of her undiagnosed trouble.

HEALING CRISIS:

When, on occasions, a worsening of the symptoms takes place, say in the alimentary tract, such as vomiting, temporary constipation, diarrhoea, etc., this often indicates that a healing process is beginning, which is never feared by those who understand the healing crisis in what is known as Nature Cure. It is rather to be looked upon as the first sign of a promising response to the treatment.

CHRONIC CONDITIONS:

The great value of the healing earth manifests itself more especially in *stubborn, chronic diseases* when the earth is taken daily over a period of some months.

Most chronic diseases, if not indeed all, are due to laziness of the bowels brought about and maintained by a long period of constipation.

ABSORPTIVE POWERS OF HEALING EARTH:

Absorption can apply equally to gases as also to fluids and solids. It is claimed that there is no other known means that so surely and permanently removes constipation than the internal use of healing earth, which can be looked upon as a food supplementing one's diet on food reform lines. Among the actions of the healing earth used EXTERNALLY in the form of compresses and packs is its absorptive quality indicated by the rapid healing of wounds, suppurations, etc.

In certain parts of Bavaria after a rainfall children have been noticed to eat the sodden earth with apparent relish, and the appearance of these children was that of radiant health. This instinctive action must have been observed by such great pioneers of Nature Cure as Priessnitz, Father Kneipp, Kühne, Rikli, Just, etc., as it is on record that some of them used earth in their healing work. Animals, too, instinctively eat the soil.

SKIN DISEASES:

On one occasion a patient asked my advice about her very valuable dog, which was afflicted with a frightful skin disease with which no vet could cope. I prescribed "Healing Clay" and after a few weeks of the dog being given this clay in its food daily and sprinkled dry on to the sores, the disease cleared up completely.

THE POWER OF THE INFINITESIMAL:

Experiment has shown that if one puts silver into distilled water and leaves it there for a few hours, this water will show a considerable biological action in that it will have a germicidal effect upon bacteria introduced into the distilled water; yet by no known method can silver be detected in the water itself. That the water HAS undergone a change is indicated by its biological action upon the bacteria.

If anyone wishes to have proof of the power of the infinitesimal dose in homoeopathy then he certainly has it in this experiment.

One estimates the attenuation of the silver in the aforementioned activated water as 30x to 40x potency. But a still greater attenuation is shown in the following example: When a glass containing the activated water is emptied and again rinsed out with distilled water and dried, and this procedure is repeated over and over again as often as one will there is always manifested in the new water the same phenomenon in that the bacteria placed in the water are killed. The glass cannot otherwise free itself from this phenomenon except by boiling with concentrated acid, e.g., nitric acid. We are here up against a secret of nature for which there is no explanation at the moment.

The action of the healing earth upon the organism belongs, to a certain extent, to the above phenomenon. For example, the fact that water that is mixed with the earth and, after it has settled, is poured off absolutely clear, will still evidence a characteristic action on a fever when applied as a compress, in that pain is more speedily removed than is the case with an ordinary Priessnitz cold water compress.

CHAPTER 34

EMETIC THERAPY

(This chapter is based mainly on the observations of Dr. Bernard Aschner)

There is an anecdote in the history of medicine that Louis IX, King of France, had been suffering from a very dangerous malignant fever. All the available medical authorities at the time had been consulted, but in vain. The King had been declared to be a hopeless case. Finally, he was abandoned to the sorcerers and charlatans. One of them, quite in accordance with an ancient doctrine, administered an emetic with the result that the King recovered within a few days.

Dr. Aschner says: "The modern physician, so greatly spoiled by too many scientific paraphernalia, instruments and gadgets, has, unfortunately 'unlearned' the mysterious ways of nature. Once upon a time the physician understood. When an attack of migraine ended with spontaneous vomiting, he rightly concluded that an emetic, given at its *onset*, would quickly prevent its development—and it does."

The unpleasant symptoms of parotitis (mumps) may often be speedily reduced by the emetics as formerly prescribed by classical medicine. This is also true in regard to ulcers of the mouth, tongue and gums, where vomiting often helps more quickly than anything else, irrespective of whether the cause is connected with the stomach or whether it is merely a case of local infection.

Medical doctors have much to learn from the veterinary surgeons, who are less influenced by changing theories, and who prefer to keep to methods that have been proved in practice, but is this so to-day? They have successfully used emetics in the past in the treatment of diphtheria in pigs. In medicine for humans, however, this powerful remedy has come to be rejected and has disappeared into oblivion. Even in very severe diphtheria of children, emetics sometimes remove the danger of suffocation and obviate the necessity of tracheotomy. The "violent" vomit clears the obstructing membranes from the upper respiratory passages and also reduces the inflammatory condition. It is because of this effect that few remedies cause TONSILLITIS to subside so quickly as an emetic.

Protection from infection can be obtained merely by the timely administration of emetics during an epidemic of whooping cough, despite direct exposure.

A physician of Reval (capital of Esthonia) once wrote a letter to Dr. Aschner, in which he stated that his five-year-old son had told him that on those days when an attack of whooping cough was accompanied by a bout of vomiting his breathing became free and his headaches ceased to trouble him. Noting this the child finally discovered a way of inducing vomiting by drinking large quantities of tea and thus found relief.

The doctor went on to ask why learned physicians lagged so far behind a child in instinctive powers of observation—why, indeed, they did everything they could to prevent the helpful vomiting process by prescribing sedatives, such as codeine and belladonna.

Hippocrates says repeatedly that unless a case of pleurisy is purged upwards by means of emetics in the early stages it may progress to pneumonia and suppuration, with its grave and often fatal results.

Most cases of pleurisy, in Europe at least, are to-day generally considered to be of tubercular origin. We wait until the exudation has reached a substantial level and then the surgeons are proud of the large quantities of fluid they are able to drain from the chest by means of syringes and other ingenious devices.

Classical medicine could, and still can, restrict and even prevent the formation of exudate at the onset, by upward and downward purging.

Vomiting has first a stimulating effect upon all the internal organs and, subsequently, a spasm-soothing one.

In states of suffocation emetics may dramatically save endangered lives even when they arise from the heart and lungs.

A physician in Talinn, another Baltic capital, some years ago, sought the advice of Dr. Aschner on behalf of his daughter, who had consulted many specialists about her bronchial asthma, but without finding any permanent relief from their treatments.

Modern remedies such as ephedrin and adrenalin and anti-allergic therapies had all been tried with only transitory results. The repeated administration of an emetic, however, together with a decoction of vegetable drugs—arnica and the roots of helenium, the classic but forgotten specifics against this disease—permanently cured the condition within a few weeks.

There is an old Sanskrit saying: "After thorough vomiting head and heart feel relieved and purged. The soul experiences a sense of well-being and serenity."

Induced vomiting is of tremendous help also in mental disease and in anxiety states. It can be looked upon as a kind of natural "shock" treatment. Overspecialised psychiatry has completely discarded this traditional and often highly effective method. Sometimes the cure succeeds almost at once, or within a few days, so that relatives and onlookers are amazed at what appears to be a "miracle," so asserts Dr. Aschner.

147

I have found that vomiting therapy is also most effective in cases of acute lumbago, as the following example will show:

A few years ago the wife of a doctor called me out to her husband as he was prostrate in bed with acute lumbago. His condition was so painful that osteopathic treatment was out of the question, his severe muscle spasm would not permit of any movement at all.

It then occurred to me to ask the doctor if he could vomit easily. "Yes" he replied, "but why?" I suggested that he drank as many glasses of water, each sweetened slightly with honey, as he could with comfort. Then he was to tickle the back of his throat with a feather or with a finger so that vomiting would be induced. This he did, he drinking a dozen glasses of water. The effect was spectacular as all the lumbar muscles lost their spasm, with the result that the doctor was free from all pain and was again quite mobile.

He told me that he had been several years in India in medical practice and had come across many "strange" methods of treatment, which worked, but never had he heard of such effectiveness of the vomiting therapy.

Besides the drinking of a few glasses of water and tickling the back of the throat to induce vomiting, herbal emetics are used, but these should be prescribed by practitioners who possess the requisite knowledge and skill in their administration. When the emetic therapy is combined with a sensible diet and other treatments that may be indicated, splendid results can be expected to follow, so that patients are seen to gain more vitality and a speedier cure.

Conditions that have been found to respond to the emetic therapy are asthma, bronchial troubles, skin diseases, throat infections, gastritis, liver and gall bladder complaints, general catarrhal conditions, acidosis, enfeebled circulation, hysteria, gangrene, eczema, psoriasis, anxiety states.

In these and other ailments the emetic treatment can lessen their severity and may be looked upon as a "short-cut" to recovery, but like every other treatment of illness it has to be judiciously employed.

If at the *very first signs* of a migraine vomiting is induced it will not develop. That is the experience of those who have tried the method.

Compton Printing Ltd., London & Aylesbury